TASTY PALEO RECIPES 2021

EASY RECIPES FOR ANY OCCASION

MELANIE BOLT

Table of Contents

4

MEXICAN SLAW

PREP: 20 minutes STAND: 2 to 4 hours MAKES: 4 servings

THERE ARE A FEW CONVENIENCE PRODUCTS THAT CAN BE INTEGRATED INTO THE PALEO DIET®—AND PACKAGED BROCCOLI SLAW IS ONE OF THEM. THE MOST COMMON TYPE IS A BLEND OF SHREDDED BROCCOLI, CARROTS, AND RED CABBAGE. IF THOSE ARE THE ONLY INGREDIENTS ON THE LABEL, FEEL FREE TO USE IT. IT CAN SAVE YOU TIME—AND WE CAN ALL USE MORE OF THAT.

1 small red onion, halved and thinly sliced

¼ cup cider vinegar

1½ cups shredded broccoli (packaged broccoli slaw)

½ cup very thin bite-size strips peeled jicama

½ cup cherry or grape tomatoes, halved

2 tablespoons snipped fresh cilantro

2 tablespoons avocado oil

1 teaspoon Mexican Seasoning (see recipe)

1 medium avocado, halved, seeded, peeled, and chopped

1. In a small bowl combine red onion and vinegar. Toss to coat. Press down on the onion slices with the back of a fork. Cover and let stand at room temperature for 2 to 4 hours, stirring occasionally.

2. In a large bowl combine broccoli, jicama, and tomatoes. Using a slotted spoon, transfer onion to the bowl with the broccoli mixture, reserving vinegar. Stir to combine.

3. For dressing, place 3 tablespoons of the reserved vinegar in a bowl (discard any remaining vinegar). Stir in cilantro, avocado oil, and Mexican Seasoning. Drizzle over broccoli mixture, tossing to coat.

4. Gently stir in avocado; serve immediately.

CREAMY CARROT AND KOHLRABI SLAW

KOHLRABI SEEMS TO BE IN THE SAME POSITION BRUSSELS SPROUTS WERE A FEW YEARS AGO—ON THE VERGE OF A RENAISSANCE DUE TO INNOVATIVE COOKS AND HEALTH-CONSCIOUS EATERS EVERYWHERE. THIS BULBOUS RELATIVE OF CABBAGE IS CRISP AND JUICY AND CAN BE EATEN RAW OR COOKED. HERE, IT'S SHREDDED AND TOSSED INTO A CRISP SLAW, BUT IT IS ALSO WONDERFUL COOKED WITH CELERY ROOT OR CARROTS AND PUREED—OR EVEN CUT INTO THICK STICKS LIKE HOME FRIES, FRIED IN OLIVE OIL, AND SEASONED WITH THE BLEND OF YOUR CHOICE (SEE "SEASONING BLENDS").

- ½ cup Paleo Mayo (see recipe)
- 2 tablespoons apple cider vinegar
- ½ teaspoon celery seeds
- ½ teaspoon paprika
- ½ teaspoon black pepper
- 2 pounds small to medium kohlrabi, peeled and coarsely shredded
- 3 medium carrots, coarsely shredded
- 1 red sweet pepper, halved, seeded, and very thinly sliced
- Snipped fresh parsley (optional)

1. In a large bowl whisk together Paleo Mayo, vinegar, celery seeds, paprika, and pepper. Gently fold in kohlrabi, carrots, and sweet pepper.

2. Cover and chill for 4 to 6 hours. Stir well before serving. If desired, sprinkle with parsley.

SMOKED BABY BACK RIBS WITH APPLE-MUSTARD MOP SAUCE

SOAK: 1 hour STAND: 15 minutes SMOKE: 4 hours COOK: 20 minutes MAKES: 4 servings PHOTO

THE RICH FLAVOR AND MEATY TEXTURE OF SMOKED RIBS CALLS FOR SOMETHING COOL AND CRISP TO GO ALONG WITH IT. ALMOST ANY SLAW WILL DO, BUT THE FENNEL SLAW (SEE RECIPE AND PICTURED HERE), IS ESPECIALLY GOOD.

RIBS
8 to 10 apple or hickory wood chunks

3 to 3½ pounds pork loin baby back ribs

¼ cup Smoky Seasoning (see recipe)

SAUCE
1 medium cooking apple, peeled, cored, and thinly sliced

¼ cup chopped onion

¼ cup water

¼ cup cider vinegar

2 tablespoons Dijon-Style Mustard (see recipe)

2 to 3 tablespoons water

1. At least 1 hour before smoke-cooking, soak wood chunks in enough water to cover. Drain before using. Trim visible fat from ribs. If necessary, peel off the thin membrane from the back of the ribs. Place ribs in a large shallow pan. Sprinkle evenly with Smoky Seasoning; rub in with your fingers. Let stand at room temperature for 15 minutes.

2. In a smoker arrange preheated coals, drained wood chunks, and water pan according to the manufacturer's directions. Pour water into pan. Place ribs, bone sides down, on grill rack over water pan. (Or place ribs in a rib rack; place rib rack on grill rack.) Cover and smoke for 2 hours. Maintain a temperature of about 225°F in the smoker for the duration of smoking. Add additional coals and water as needed to maintain temperature and moisture.

3. Meanwhile, for mop sauce, in a small saucepan combine apple slices, onion, and the ¼ cup water. Bring to boiling; reduce heat. Simmer, covered, for 10 to 12 minutes or until apple slices are very tender, stirring occasionally. Cool slightly; transfer undrained apple and onion to a food processor or blender. Cover and process or blend until smooth. Return puree to saucepan. Stir in vinegar and Dijon-Style Mustard. Cook over medium-low heat for 5 minutes, stirring occasionally. Add 2 to 3 tablespoons of water (or more, as needed) to make the sauce the consistency of a vinaigrette. Divide the sauce into thirds.

4. After 2 hours, brush ribs generously with one-third of the mop sauce. Cover and smoke 1 hour more. Brush again with another one-third of the mop sauce. Wrap each slab of ribs in heavy foil and place the ribs back on the smoker, layering them on top of each other if needed. Cover and smoke for 1 to 1½ hours more or until ribs are tender.*

5. Unwrap ribs and brush with the remaining one-third of the mop sauce. Cut ribs between bones to serve.

*Tip: To test tenderness of the ribs, carefully remove the foil from one of the slabs of ribs. Pick up the rib slab with tongs, holding the slab by the top one-fourth of the slab. Turn the rib slab over so the meaty side is facing down. If the ribs are tender, the slab should begin to fall apart as you pick it up. If it is not tender, wrap again in foil and continue to smoke ribs until tender.

OVEN BBQ COUNTRY-STYLE PORK RIBS WITH FRESH PINEAPPLE SLAW

PREP: 20 minutes COOK: 8 minutes BAKE: 1 hour 15 minutes MAKES: 4 servings

COUNTRY-STYLE PORK RIBS ARE MEATY, INEXPENSIVE, AND, IF TREATED THE RIGHT WAY—SUCH AS COOKED LOW AND SLOW IN A MESS OF BARBECUE SAUCE—GET MELTINGLY TENDER.

2 pounds boneless country-style pork ribs

¼ teaspoon black pepper

1 tablespoon refined coconut oil

½ cup fresh orange juice

1½ cups BBQ Sauce (see recipe)

3 cups shredded green and/or red cabbage

1 cup shredded carrots

2 cups finely chopped pineapple

⅓ cup Bright Citrus Vinaigrette (see recipe)

BBQ Sauce (see recipe) (optional)

1. Preheat oven to 350°F. Sprinkle pork with pepper. In an extra-large skillet heat coconut oil over medium-high heat. Add pork ribs; cook for 8 to 10 minutes or until browned, turning to brown evenly. Place ribs in a 3-quart rectangular baking dish.

2. For sauce, add orange juice to skillet, stirring to scrape up any browned bits. Stir in the 1½ cups BBQ Sauce. Pour sauce over ribs. Turn ribs to coat with sauce (if necessary, use a pastry brush to brush sauce over ribs). Cover baking dish tightly with aluminum foil.

13

3. Bake ribs for 1 hour. Remove foil and brush ribs with sauce from baking dish. Bake about 15 minutes more or until ribs are tender and browned and sauce has thickened slightly.

4. Meanwhile, for pineapple slaw, combine cabbage, carrots, pineapple, and Bright Citrus Vinaigrette. Cover and refrigerate until serving time.

5. Serve ribs with slaw and, if desired, additional BBQ Sauce.

SPICY PORK GOULASH

PREP: 20 minutes COOK: 40 minutes MAKES: 6 servings

THIS HUNGARIAN-STYLE STEW IS SERVED ON A BED OF CRUNCHY, BARELY WILTED CABBAGE FOR A ONE-DISH MEAL. CRUSH THE CARAWAY SEEDS IN A MORTAR AND PESTLE IF YOU HAVE ONE. IF NOT, CRUSH THEM UNDER THE BROAD SIDE OF A CHEF'S KNIFE BY PRESSING DOWN ON KNIFE GENTLY WITH YOUR FIST.

GOULASH

- 1½ pounds ground pork
- 2 cups chopped red, orange, and/or yellow sweet peppers
- ¾ cup finely chopped red onion
- 1 small fresh red chile, seeded and finely chopped (see tip)
- 4 teaspoons Smoky Seasoning (see recipe)
- 1 teaspoon caraway seeds, crushed
- ¼ teaspoon ground marjoram or oregano
- 1 14-ounce can no-salt-added diced tomatoes, undrained
- 2 tablespoons red wine vinegar
- 1 tablespoon finely shredded lemon peel
- ⅓ cup snipped fresh parsley

CABBAGE

- 2 tablespoons olive oil
- 1 medium onion, sliced
- 1 small head green or red cabbage, cored and thinly sliced

1. For the goulash, in a large Dutch oven cook ground pork, sweet peppers, and onion over medium-high heat for 8 to 10 minutes or until the pork is no longer pink and vegetables are crisp-tender, stirring with a wooden spoon to break up meat. Drain off fat. Reduce heat to

low; add red chile, Smoky Seasoning, caraway seeds, and marjoram. Cover and cook for 10 minutes. Add undrained tomatoes and vinegar. Bring to boiling; reduce heat. Simmer, covered, for 20 minutes.

2. Meanwhile, for cabbage, in an extra-large skillet heat oil over medium heat. Add onion and cook until softened, about 2 minutes. Add cabbage; stir to combine. Reduce heat to low. Cook about 8 minutes or until cabbage is just tender, stirring occasionally.

3. To serve, place some of the cabbage mixture on a plate. Top with goulash and sprinkle with lemon zest and parsley.

ITALIAN SAUSAGE MEATBALLS MARINARA WITH SLICED FENNEL AND ONION SAUTÉ

PREP: 30 minutes BAKE: 30 minutes COOK: 40 minutes MAKES: 4 to 6 servings

THIS RECIPE IS A RARE EXAMPLE OF A CANNED PRODUCT WORKING AS WELL AS—IF NOT BETTER THAN—THE FRESH VERSION. UNLESS YOU HAVE TOMATOES THAT ARE VERY, VERY RIPE, YOU WILL NOT GET AS GOOD A CONSISTENCY IN A SAUCE USING FRESH TOMATOES AS YOU CAN USING CANNED TOMATOES. JUST BE SURE YOU USE A NO-SALT-ADDED PRODUCT— AND, EVEN BETTER, ORGANIC.

MEATBALLS

- 2 large eggs
- ½ cup almond meal
- 8 cloves garlic, minced
- 6 tablespoons dry white wine
- 1 tablespoon paprika
- 2 teaspoons black pepper
- 1 teaspoon fennel seeds, lightly crushed
- 1 teaspoon dried oregano, crushed
- 1 teaspoon dried thyme, crushed
- ¼ to ½ teaspoon cayenne pepper
- 1½ pounds ground pork

MARINARA

- 2 tablespoons olive oil
- 2 15-ounce cans no-salt-added crushed tomatoes or one 28-ounce can no-salt-added crushed tomatoes
- ½ cup snipped fresh basil

17

3 medium fennel bulbs, halved, cored, and thinly sliced

1 large sweet onion, halved and thinly sliced

1. Preheat oven to 375°F. Line a large rimmed baking sheet with parchment paper; set aside. In a large bowl whisk together the eggs, almond meal, 6 cloves of the minced garlic, 3 tablespoons of the wine, the paprika, 1½ teaspoons of the black pepper, the fennel seeds, oregano, thyme, and cayenne pepper. Add the pork; mix well. Shape pork mixture into 1½-inch meatballs (should have about 24 meatballs); arrange in a single layer on the prepared baking sheet. Bake about 30 minutes or until lightly browned, turning once while baking.

2. Meanwhile, for marinara sauce, in a 4- to 6-quart Dutch oven heat 1 tablespoon of the olive oil. Add the 2 remaining cloves minced garlic; cook about 1 minute or until just starting to brown. Quickly add the remaining 3 tablespoons wine, the crushed tomatoes, and the basil. Bring to boiling; reduce heat. Simmer, uncovered, for 5 minutes. Carefully stir the cooked meatballs into the marinara sauce. Cover and simmer for 25 to 30 minutes.

3. Meanwhile, in a large skillet heat the remaining 1 tablespoon olive oil over medium heat. Stir in the sliced fennel and onion. Cook for 8 to 10 minutes or until just tender and lightly browned, stirring frequently. Season with the remaining ½ teaspoon black pepper. Serve the meatballs and marinara sauce over the fennel and onion sauté.

PORK-STUFFED ZUCCHINI BOATS WITH BASIL AND PINE NUTS

PREP: 20 minutes COOK: 22 minutes BAKE: 20 minutes MAKES: 4 servings

KIDS WILL LOVE THIS FUN-TO-EAT DISH OF HOLLOWED-OUT ZUCCHINI STUFFED WITH GROUND PORK, TOMATOES, AND SWEET PEPPERS. IF YOU LIKE, STIR IN 3 TABLESPOONS OF BASIL PESTO (SEE RECIPE) IN PLACE OF THE FRESH BASIL, PARSLEY, AND PINE NUTS.

2 medium zucchini

1 tablespoon extra virgin olive oil

12 ounces ground pork

¾ cup chopped onion

2 cloves garlic, minced

1 cup chopped tomatoes

⅔ cup finely chopped yellow or orange sweet pepper

1 teaspoon fennel seeds, lightly crushed

½ teaspoon crushed red pepper flakes

¼ cup snipped fresh basil

3 tablespoons snipped fresh parsley

2 tablespoons pine nuts, toasted (see tip) and coarsely chopped

1 teaspoon finely shredded lemon peel

1. Preheat oven to 350°F. Halve zucchini lengthwise and carefully scrape out the center, leaving ¼-inch-thick shell. Coarsely chop the zucchini pulp and set aside. Arrange zucchini halves, cut sides up, on a foil-lined baking sheet.

2. For filling, in a large skillet heat the olive oil over medium-high heat. Add ground pork; cook until no longer pink, stirring with a wooden spoon to break up meat. Drain off

19

fat. Reduce heat to medium. Add the reserved zucchini pulp, onion, and garlic; cook and stir about 8 minutes or until onion is soft. Stir in the tomatoes, sweet pepper, fennel seeds, and crushed red pepper. Cook about 10 minutes or until tomatoes are soft and beginning to break down. Remove pan from heat. Stir in the basil, parsley, pine nuts, and lemon peel. Divide filling among zucchini shells, mounding slightly. Bake for 20 to 25 minutes or until zucchini shells are crisp-tender.

CURRIED PORK AND PINEAPPLE "NOODLE" BOWLS WITH COCONUT MILK AND HERBS

PREP: 30 minutes COOK: 15 minutes BAKE: 40 minutes MAKES: 4 servings PHOTO

1 large spaghetti squash

2 tablespoons refined coconut oil

1 pound ground pork

2 tablespoons finely chopped scallions

2 tablespoons fresh lime juice

1 tablespoon minced fresh ginger

6 cloves garlic, minced

1 tablespoon minced lemongrass

1 tablespoon no-salt-added Thai-style red curry powder

1 cup chopped red sweet pepper

1 cup chopped onion

½ cup julienne-cut carrot

1 baby bok choy, sliced (3 cups)

1 cup sliced fresh button mushrooms

1 or 2 Thai bird chiles, thinly sliced (see tip)

1 13.5-ounce can natural coconut milk (such as Nature's Way)

½ cup Chicken Bone Broth (see recipe) or no-salt-added chicken broth

¼ cup fresh pineapple juice

3 tablespoons unsalted no-oil-added cashew butter

1 cup cubed fresh pineapple, cubed

Lime wedges

Fresh cilantro, mint, and/or Thai basil

Chopped roasted cashews

1. Preheat oven to 400°F. Microwave spaghetti squash on high for 3 minutes. Carefully cut the squash in half

lengthwise and scrape out the seeds. Rub 1 tablespoon of the coconut oil over the cut sides of the squash. Place squash halves, cut sides down, on a baking sheet. Bake for 40 to 50 minutes or until squash can be pierced easily with a knife. Using the tines of a fork, scrape the flesh from the shells and keep warm until ready to serve.

2. Meanwhile, in a medium bowl combine the pork, scallions, lime juice, ginger, garlic, lemongrass, and curry powder; mix well. In an extra-large skillet heat the remaining 1 tablespoon of the coconut oil over medium-high heat. Add pork mixture; cook until no longer pink, stirring with a wooden spoon to break up meat. Add the sweet pepper, onion, and carrot; cook and stir about 3 minutes or until vegetables are crisp-tender. Stir in the bok choy, mushrooms, chiles, coconut milk, Chicken Bone Broth, pineapple juice, and cashew butter. Bring to boiling; reduce heat. Add pineapple; simmer, uncovered, until heated through.

3. To serve, divide the spaghetti squash among four serving bowls. Ladle the curried pork over the squash. Serve with lime wedges, herbs, and cashews.

SPICY GRILLED PORK PATTIES WITH TANGY CUCUMBER SALAD

PREP: 30 minutes GRILL: 10 minutes STAND: 10 minutes MAKES: 4 servings

THE CRUNCHY CUCUMBER SALAD FLAVORED WITH FRESH MINT IS A COOLING AND REFRESHING COMPLEMENT TO THE SPICY PORK BURGERS.

⅓ cup olive oil

¼ cup chopped fresh mint

3 tablespoons white wine vinegar

8 cloves garlic, minced

¼ teaspoon black pepper

2 medium cucumbers, very thinly sliced

1 small onion, cut into thin slivers (about ½ cup)

1¼ to 1½ pounds ground pork

¼ cup chopped fresh cilantro

1 to 2 medium fresh jalapeño or serrano chile peppers, seeded (if desired) and finely chopped (see tip)

2 medium red sweet peppers, seeded and quartered

2 teaspoons olive oil

1. In a large bowl whisk together ⅓ cup olive oil, mint, vinegar, 2 cloves minced garlic, and the black pepper. Add sliced cucumbers and onion. Toss until well coated. Cover and chill until ready to serve, stirring once or twice.

2. In a large bowl combine pork, cilantro, chile pepper, and the remaining 6 cloves minced garlic. Shape into four ¾-inch-thick patties. Brush pepper quarters lightly with the 2 teaspoons olive oil.

23

3. For a charcoal or gas grill, place patties and sweet pepper quarters directly over medium heat. Cover and grill until an instant-read thermometer inserted into sides of pork patties registers 160°F and pepper quarters are tender and lightly charred, turning patties and pepper quarters once halfway through grilling. Allow 10 to 12 minutes for patties and 8 to 10 minutes for the pepper quarters.

4. When pepper quarters are done, wrap them in a piece of foil to completely enclose. Let stand about 10 minutes or until cool enough to handle. Using a sharp knife, carefully peel off the pepper skins. Thinly slice pepper quarters lengthwise.

5. To serve, stir cucumber salad and spoon evenly onto four large serving plates. Add a pork patty to each plate. Pile the red pepper slices evenly on top of patties.

ZUCCHINI-CRUST PIZZA WITH SUN-DRIED TOMATO PESTO, SWEET PEPPERS, AND ITALIAN SAUSAGE

PREP: 30 minutes COOK: 15 minutes BAKE: 30 minutes MAKES: 4 servings

THIS IS KNIFE-AND-FORK PIZZA. BE SURE TO PRESS THE SAUSAGE AND PEPPERS LIGHTLY INTO THE PESTO-COATED CRUST SO THAT THE TOPPINGS ADHERE ENOUGH FOR THE PIZZA TO CUT NEATLY.

2 tablespoons olive oil

1 tablespoon finely ground almonds

1 large egg, lightly beaten

½ cup almond flour

1 tablespoon snipped fresh oregano

¼ teaspoon black pepper

3 cloves garlic, minced

3½ cups shredded zucchini (2 medium)

Italian Sausage (see recipe, below)

1 tablespoon extra virgin olive oil

1 sweet pepper (yellow, red, or half of each), seeded and cut into very thin strips

1 small onion, thinly sliced

Sun-Dried Tomato Pesto (see recipe, below)

1. Preheat oven to 425°F. Brush a 12-inch pizza pan with the 2 tablespoons olive oil. Sprinkle with ground almonds; set aside.

2. For crust, in a large bowl combine egg, almond flour, oregano, black pepper, and garlic. Place shredded

25

zucchini in a clean towel or piece of cheesecloth. Wrap tightly

SMOKED LEMON-CORIANDER LAMB LEG WITH GRILLED ASPARAGUS

SOAK: 30 minutes PREP: 20 minutes GRILL: 45 minutes STAND: 10 minutes
MAKES: 6 to 8 servings

SIMPLE BUT ELEGANT, THIS DISH FEATURES TWO INGREDIENTS THAT COME INTO THEIR OWN IN THE SPRING—LAMB AND ASPARAGUS. TOASTING THE CORIANDER SEEDS ENHANCES THE WARM, EARTHY, SLIGHTLY TANGY FLAVOR.

1 cup hickory wood chips

2 tablespoons coriander seeds

2 tablespoons finely shredded lemon peel

1½ teaspoons black pepper

2 tablespoons snipped fresh thyme

1 2- to 3-pound boneless leg of lamb

2 bunches fresh asparagus

1 tablespoon olive oil

¼ teaspoon black pepper

1 lemon, cut into quarters

1. At least 30 minutes before smoke-cooking, in a bowl soak hickory chips in enough water to cover; set aside. Meanwhile, in a small skillet toast coriander seeds over medium heat about 2 minutes or until fragrant and crackling, stirring frequently. Remove seeds from skillet; let cool. When seeds have cooled, coarsely crush in a mortar and pestle (or place seeds on a cutting board and crush them with the back of a wooden spoon). In a

small bowl combine crushed coriander seeds, lemon peel, the 1½ teaspoons pepper, and thyme; set aside.

2. Remove netting from lamb roast if present. On a work surface open up the roast, fat side down. Sprinkle half of the spice mixture over meat; rub in with your fingers. Roll the roast up and tie with four to six pieces of 100%-cotton kitchen string. Sprinkle the remaining spice mixture over outside of roast, pressing lightly to adhere.

3. For a charcoal grill, arrange medium-hot coals around a drip pan. Test for medium heat above the pan. Sprinkle the drained wood chips over the coals. Place lamb roast on the grill rack over the drip pan. Cover and smoke for 40 to 50 minutes for medium (145°F). (For a gas grill, preheat grill. Reduce heat to medium. Adjust for indirect cooking. Smoke as above, except add drained wood chips according to manufacturer's directions.) Cover roast loosely with foil. Let stand for 10 minutes before slicing.

4. Meanwhile, trim woody ends from asparagus. In a large bowl toss asparagus with olive oil and the ¼ teaspoon pepper. Place asparagus around outer edges of grill, directly over the coals and perpendicular to the grill grate. Cover and grill for 5 to 6 minutes until crisp-tender. Squeeze lemon wedges over asparagus.

5. Remove string from lamb roast and thinly slice meat. Serve meat with grilled asparagus.

LAMB HOT POT

PREP: 30 minutes COOK: 2 hours 40 minutes MAKES: 4 servings

WARM UP WITH THIS SAVORY STEW ON A FALL OR WINTER NIGHT. THE STEW IS SERVED OVER A VELVETY CELERY ROOT-PARSNIP MASH FLAVORED WITH DIJON-STYLE MUSTARD, CASHEW CREAM, AND CHIVES. NOTE: CELERY ROOT IS SOMETIMES CALLED CELERIAC.

- 10 black peppercorns
- 6 sage leaves
- 3 whole allspice
- 2 2-inch strips orange peel
- 2 pounds boneless lamb shoulder
- 3 tablespoons olive oil
- 2 medium onions, coarsely chopped
- 1 14.5-ounce can no-salt-added diced tomatoes, undrained
- 1½ cups Beef Bone Broth (see recipe) or no-salt-added beef broth
- ¾ cup dry white wine
- 3 large cloves garlic, crushed and peeled
- 2 pounds celery root, peeled and cut into 1-inch cubes
- 6 medium parsnips, peeled and cut into 1-inch slices (about 2 pounds)
- 2 tablespoons olive oil
- 2 tablespoons Cashew Cream (see recipe)
- 1 tablespoon Dijon-Style Mustard (see recipe)
- ¼ cup snipped chives

1. For the bouquet garni, cut a 7-inch square of cheesecloth. Place peppercorns, sage, allspice, and orange peel in center of cheesecloth. Bring up the corners of the cheesecloth and tie securely with clean 100%-cotton kitchen string. Set aside.

2. Trim fat from lamb shoulder; cut lamb into 1-inch pieces. In a Dutch oven heat the 3 tablespoons olive oil over medium heat. Cook lamb, in batches if necessary, in hot oil until browned; remove from pan and keep warm. Add onions to pan; cook for 5 to 8 minutes or until softened and lightly browned. Add bouquet garni, undrained tomatoes, 1¼ cups of the Beef Bone Broth, wine, and garlic. Bring to boiling; reduce heat. Simmer, covered, for 2 hours, stirring occasionally. Remove and discard bouquet garni.

3. Meanwhile, for mash, place celery root and parsnips in a large stockpot; cover with water. Bring to boiling over medium-high heat; reduce heat to low. Cover and simmer gently for 30 to 40 minutes or until the vegetables are very tender when pierced with a fork. Drain; place vegetables in a food processor. Add the remaining ¼ cup Beef Bone Broth and the 2 tablespoons oil; pulse until mash is almost smooth but still has some texture, stopping once or twice to scrape down the sides. Transfer mash to a bowl. Stir in Cashew Cream, mustard, and chives.

4. To serve, divide mash among four bowls; top with Lamb Hot Pot.

LAMB STEW WITH CELERY-ROOT NOODLES

PREP: 30 minutes BAKE: 1 hour 30 minutes MAKES: 6 servings

CELERY ROOT TAKES AN ENTIRELY DIFFERENT FORM IN THIS STEW THAN IT DOES IN THE LAMB HOT POT (SEE RECIPE). A MANDOLINE SLICER IS USED TO CREATE VERY THIN STRIPS OF THE SWEET AND NUTTY-TASTING ROOT. THE "NOODLES" SIMMER IN THE STEW UNTIL THEY ARE TENDER.

- 2 teaspoons Lemon-Herb Seasoning (see recipe)
- 1½ pounds lamb stew meat, cut into 1-inch cubes
- 2 tablespoons olive oil
- 2 cups chopped onions
- 1 cup chopped carrots
- 1 cup diced turnips
- 1 tablespoon minced garlic (6 cloves)
- 2 tablespoons no-salt-added tomato paste
- ½ cup dry red wine
- 4 cups Beef Bone Broth (see recipe) or no-salt-added beef broth
- 1 bay leaf
- 2 cups 1-inch cubes butternut squash
- 1 cup diced eggplant
- 1 pound celery root, peeled
- Chopped fresh parsley

1. Preheat oven to 250°F. Sprinkle Lemon-Herb Seasoning evenly over lamb. Toss gently to coat. Heat a 6- to 8-quart Dutch oven over medium-high heat. Add 1 tablespoon of the olive oil and half of the seasoned lamb to the Dutch oven. Brown meat in hot oil on all

31

sides; transfer browned meat to a plate and repeat with remaining lamb and olive oil. Reduce heat to medium.

2. Add onions, carrots, and turnips to pot. Cook and stir vegetables for 4 minutes; add garlic and tomato paste and cook 1 minute more. Add red wine, Beef Bone Broth, bay leaf, and reserved meat and any accumulated juices to pot. Bring mixture to a simmer. Cover and place Dutch oven in preheated oven. Bake for 1 hour. Stir in butternut squash and eggplant. Return to oven and bake for an additional 30 minutes.

3. While stew is in oven, use a mandoline to very thinly slice celery root. Cut celery root slices into ½-inch-wide strips. (You should have about 4 cups.) Stir celery root strips into stew. Simmer about 10 minutes or until tender. Remove and discard bay leaf before serving stew. Sprinkle each serving with chopped parsley.

FRENCHED LAMB CHOPS WITH POMEGRANATE-DATE CHUTNEY

PREP: 10 minutes COOK: 18 minutes COOL: 10 minutes MAKES: 4 servings

THE TERM "FRENCHED" REFERS TO A RIB BONE FROM WHICH FAT, MEAT, AND CONNECTIVE TISSUE HAVE BEEN REMOVED WITH A SHARP PARING KNIFE. IT MAKES FOR AN ATTRACTIVE PRESENTATION. ASK YOUR BUTCHER TO DO IT OR YOU CAN DO IT YOURSELF.

CHUTNEY

½ cup unsweetened pomegranate juice

1 tablespoon fresh lemon juice

1 shallot, peeled and thinly sliced into rings

1 teaspoon finely shredded orange peel

⅓ cup chopped Medjool dates

¼ teaspoon crushed red pepper

¼ cup pomegranate arils*

1 tablespoon olive oil

1 tablespoon chopped fresh Italian (flat-leaf) parsley

LAMB CHOPS

2 tablespoons olive oil

8 frenched lamb rib chops

1. For the chutney, in a small skillet combine pomegranate juice, lemon juice, and shallot. Bring to boiling; reduce heat. Simmer, uncovered, for 2 minutes. Add orange peel, dates, and crushed red pepper. Let stand until cool, about 10 minutes. Stir in pomegranate arils, the 1 tablespoon olive oil, and the parsley. Set aside at room temperature until serving time.

33

2. For the chops, in a large skillet heat the 2 tablespoons olive oil over medium heat. Working in batches, add chops to skillet and cook for 6 to 8 minutes for medium rare (145°F), turning once. Top chops with chutney.

*Note: Fresh pomegranates and their arils, or seeds, are available from October through February. If you can't find them, use unsweetened dried seeds to add crunch to the chutney.

CHIMICHURRI LAMB LOIN CHOPS WITH SAUTÉED RADICCHIO SLAW

PREP: 30 minutes MARINATE: 20 minutes COOK: 20 minutes MAKES: 4 servings

IN ARGENTINA, CHIMICHURRI IS THE MOST POPULAR CONDIMENT ACCOMPANYING THAT COUNTRY'S RENOWNED GAUCHO-STYLE GRILLED STEAK. THERE ARE LOTS OF VARIATIONS, BUT THE THICK HERB SAUCE IS USUALLY BUILT AROUND PARSLEY, CILANTRO OR OREGANO, SHALLOTS AND/OR GARLIC, CRUSHED RED PEPPER, OLIVE OIL, AND RED WINE VINEGAR. IT'S GREAT ON GRILLED STEAK BUT EQUALLY BRILLIANT ON ROASTED OR PAN-SEARED LAMB CHOPS, CHICKEN, AND PORK.

8 lamb loin chops, cut 1 inch thick

½ cup Chimichurri Sauce (see recipe)

2 tablespoons olive oil

1 sweet onion, halved and sliced

1 teaspoon cumin seeds, crushed*

1 clove garlic, minced

1 head radicchio, cored and sliced into thin ribbons

1 tablespoon balsamic vinegar

1. Place lamb chops in an extra-large bowl. Drizzle with 2 tablespoons of the Chimichurri Sauce. Using your fingers, rub the sauce over the entire surface of each chop. Let chops marinate at room temperature for 20 minutes.

2. Meanwhile, for sautéed radicchio slaw, in an extra-large skillet heat 1 tablespoon of the olive oil. Add onion,

cumin seeds, and garlic; cook for 6 to 7 minutes or until onion softens, stirring frequently. Add radicchio; cook for 1 to 2 minutes or until radicchio just wilts slightly. Transfer slaw to a large bowl. Add balsamic vinegar and toss well to combine. Cover and keep warm.

3. Wipe out skillet. Add the remaining 1 tablespoon olive oil to the skillet and heat over medium-high heat. Add the lamb chops; reduce heat to medium. Cook for 9 to 11 minutes or until desired doneness, turning chops occasionally with tongs.

4. Serve chops with slaw and the remaining Chimichurri Sauce.

*Note: To crush cumin seeds, use a mortar and pestle—or place seeds on a cutting board and crush with a chef's knife.

ANCHO-AND-SAGE-RUBBED LAMB CHOPS WITH CARROT-SWEET POTATO REMOULADE

PREP: 12 minutes CHILL: 1 to 2 hours GRILL: 6 minutes MAKES: 4 servings

THERE ARE THREE TYPES OF LAMB CHOPS. THICK AND MEATY LOIN CHOPS LOOK LIKE SMALL T-BONE STEAKS. RIB CHOPS—CALLED FOR HERE—ARE CREATED BY CUTTING BETWEEN THE BONES OF A RACK OF LAMB. THEY ARE VERY TENDER AND HAVE A LONG, ATTRACTIVE BONE ON THE SIDE. THEY ARE OFTEN SERVED PAN-SEARED OR GRILLED. BUDGET-FRIENDLY SHOULDER CHOPS ARE A BIT FATTIER AND LESS TENDER THAN THE OTHER TWO TYPES. THEY ARE BEST BROWNED AND THEN BRAISED IN WINE, STOCK, AND TOMATOES—OR SOME COMBINATION OF THEM.

3 medium carrots, coarsely shredded

2 small sweet potatoes, julienne-cut* or coarsely shredded

½ cup Paleo Mayo (see recipe)

2 tablespoons fresh lemon juice

2 teaspoons Dijon-Style Mustard (see recipe)

2 tablespoons snipped fresh parsley

½ teaspoon black pepper

8 lamb rib chops, cut ½ to ¾ inch thick

2 tablespoon snipped fresh sage or 2 teaspoons dried sage, crushed

2 teaspoons ground ancho chile pepper

½ teaspoon garlic powder

1. For the remoulade, in a medium bowl combine carrots and sweet potatoes. In a small bowl stir together Paleo Mayo, lemon juice, Dijon-Style Mustard, parsley, and

black pepper. Pour over carrots and sweet potatoes; toss to coat. Cover and chill for 1 to 2 hours.

2. Meanwhile, in a small bowl combine sage, ancho chile, and garlic powder. Rub spice mixture onto lamb chops.

3. For a charcoal or gas grill, place lamb chops on a grill rack directly over medium heat. Cover and grill for 6 to 8 minutes for medium rare (145°F) or 10 to 12 minutes for medium (150°F), turning once halfway through grilling.

4. Serve the lamb chops with the remoulade.

*Note: Use a mandoline with a julienne attachment to cut the sweet potatoes.

LAMB CHOPS WITH SHALLOT, MINT, AND OREGANO RUB

PREP: 20 minutes MARINATE: 1 to 24 hours ROAST: 40 minutes GRILL: 12 minutes
MAKES: 4 servings

AS WITH MOST MARINATED MEATS, THE LONGER YOU LEAVE THE HERB RUB ON THE LAMB CHOPS BEFORE COOKING, THE MORE FLAVORFUL THEY WILL BE. THERE IS AN EXCEPTION TO THIS RULE, AND THAT IS WHEN YOU ARE USING A MARINADE THAT CONTAINS HIGHLY ACIDIC INGREDIENTS SUCH AS CITRUS JUICE, VINEGAR, AND WINE. IF YOU LET THE MEAT SIT IN AN ACIDIC MARINADE TOO LONG, IT BEGINS TO BREAK DOWN AND GET MUSHY.

LAMB

- 2 tablespoons finely chopped shallot
- 2 tablespoons finely chopped fresh mint
- 2 tablespoons finely chopped fresh oregano
- 5 teaspoons Mediterranean Seasoning (see recipe)
- 4 teaspoons olive oil
- 2 cloves garlic, minced
- 8 lamb rib chops, cut about 1 inch thick

SALAD

- ¾ pound baby beets, trimmed
- 1 tablespoon olive oil
- ¼ cup fresh lemon juice
- ¼ cup olive oil
- 1 tablespoon finely chopped shallot
- 1 teaspoon Dijon-Style Mustard (see recipe)
- 6 cups mixed greens
- 4 teaspoons snipped chives

1. For the lamb, in a small bowl combine 2 tablespoons shallot, mint, oregano, 4 teaspoons of the Mediterranean seasoning, and 4 teaspoons olive oil. Sprinkle rub over all sides of the lamb chops; rub in with your fingers. Place chops on a plate; cover with plastic wrap and refrigerate for at least 1 hour or up to 24 hours to marinate.

2. For salad, preheat oven to 400°F. Scrub beets well; cut into wedges. Place in a 2-quart baking dish. Drizzle with the 1 tablespoon olive oil. Cover dish with foil. Roast about 40 minutes or until beets are tender. Cool completely. (Beets can be roasted up to 2 days ahead.)

3. In a screw-top jar combine lemon juice, ¼ cup olive oil, 1 tablespoon shallot, Dijon-Style Mustard, and the remaining 1 teaspoon Mediterranean Seasoning. Cover and shake well. In a salad bowl combine beets and greens; toss with some of the vinaigrette.

4. For a charcoal or gas grill, place chops on the greased grill rack directly over medium heat. Cover and grill to desired doneness, turning once halfway through grilling. Allow 12 to 14 minutes for medium rare (145°F) or 15 to 17 minutes for medium (160°F).

5. To serve, place 2 lamb chops and some of the salad on each of four serving plates. Sprinkle with chives. Pass remaining vinaigrette.

GARDEN-STUFFED LAMB BURGERS WITH RED PEPPER COULIS

PREP: 20 minutes STAND: 15 minutes GRILL: 27 minutes MAKES: 4 servings

A COULIS IS NOTHING MORE THAN A SIMPLE, SMOOTH SAUCE MADE FROM PUREED FRUITS OR VEGETABLES. THE BRIGHT AND BEAUTIFUL RED PEPPER SAUCE FOR THESE LAMB BURGERS GETS A DOUBLE DOSE OF SMOKE—FROM GRILLING AND FROM A SHOT OF SMOKED PAPRIKA.

RED PEPPER COULIS

- 1 large red sweet pepper
- 1 tablespoon dry white wine or white wine vinegar
- 1 teaspoon olive oil
- ½ teaspoon smoked paprika

BURGERS

- ¼ cup snipped unsulfured dried tomatoes
- ¼ cup shredded zucchini
- 1 tablespoon snipped fresh basil
- 2 teaspoons olive oil
- ½ teaspoon black pepper
- 1½ pounds ground lamb
- 1 egg white, lightly beaten
- 1 tablespoon Mediterranean Seasoning (see recipe)

1. For the red pepper coulis, place the red pepper on the grill rack directly over medium heat. Cover and grill for 15 to 20 minutes or until charred and very tender, turning the pepper about every 5 minutes to char each

41

side. Remove from the grill and immediately place in a paper bag or foil to completely enclose the pepper. Let stand for 15 minutes or until cool enough to handle. Using a sharp knife, gently pull off skins and discard. Quarter pepper lengthwise and remove stems, seeds, and membranes. In a food processor combine the roasted pepper, wine, olive oil, and smoked paprika. Cover and process or blend until smooth.

2. Meanwhile, for the filling, place dried tomatoes in a small bowl and cover with boiling water. Let stand for 5 minutes; drain. Pat tomatoes and shredded zucchini dry with paper towels. In the small bowl stir together tomatoes, zucchini, basil, olive oil, and ¼ teaspoon of the black pepper; set aside.

3. In a large bowl combine ground lamb, egg white, remaining ¼ teaspoon black pepper, and Mediterranean Seasoning; mix well. Divide meat mixture into eight equal portions and shape each into a ¼-inch-thick patty. Spoon filling onto four of the patties; top with remaining patties and pinch edges to seal in the filling.

4. Place patties on the grill rack directly over medium heat. Cover and grill for 12 to 14 minutes or until done (160°F), turning once halfway through grilling.

5. To serve, top burgers with red pepper coulis.

DOUBLE-OREGANO LAMB KABOBS WITH TZATZIKI SAUCE

SOAK: 30 minutes PREP: 20 minutes CHILL: 30 minutes GRILL: 8 minutes MAKES: 4 servings

THESE LAMB KABOBS ARE ESSENTIALLY WHAT IS KNOWN AS KOFTA IN THE MEDITERRANEAN AND MIDDLE EAST—SEASONED GROUND MEAT (USUALLY LAMB OR BEEF) IS SHAPED INTO BALLS OR AROUND A SKEWER AND THEN GRILLED. FRESH AND DRIED OREGANO GIVE THEM GREAT GREEK FLAVOR.

8 10-inch wooden skewers

LAMB KABOBS

1½ pounds lean ground lamb

1 small onion, shredded and squeezed dry

1 tablespoon snipped fresh oregano

2 teaspoon dried oregano, crushed

1 teaspoon black pepper

TZATZIKI SAUCE

1 cup Paleo Mayo (see recipe)

½ of a large cucumber, seeded and shredded and squeezed dry

2 tablespoons fresh lemon juice

1 clove garlic, minced

1. Soak skewers in enough water to cover for 30 minutes.

2. For lamb kabobs, in a large bowl combine ground lamb, onion, fresh and dried oregano, and pepper; mix well. Divide the lamb mixture into eight equal portions. Shape each portion around half of a skewer, creating a 5×1-inch log. Cover and chill for at least 30 minutes.

43

3. Meanwhile, for Tzatziki Sauce, in a small bowl combine Paleo Mayo, cucumber, lemon juice, and garlic. Cover and chill until serving.

4. For a charcoal or gas grill, place lamb kabobs on grill rack directly over medium heat. Cover and grill about 8 minutes for medium (160°F), turning once halfway through grilling.

5. Serve lamb kabobs with Tzatziki Sauce.

ROAST CHICKEN WITH SAFFRON AND LEMON

PREP: 15 minutes CHILL: 8 hours ROAST: 1 hour 15 minutes STAND: 10 minutes
MAKES: 4 servings

SAFFRON IS THE DRIED STAMENS OF A TYPE OF CROCUS FLOWER. IT IS PRICEY, BUT A LITTLE GOES A LONG WAY. IT ADDS ITS EARTHY, DISTINCTIVE FLAVOR AND GORGEOUS YELLOW HUE TO THIS CRISP-SKINNED ROAST CHICKEN.

1 4- to 5-pound whole chicken

3 tablespoons olive oil

6 cloves garlic, crushed and peeled

1½ tablespoons finely shredded lemon peel

1 tablespoon fresh thyme

1½ teaspoons cracked black pepper

½ teaspoon saffron threads

2 bay leaves

1 lemon, quartered

1. Remove neck and giblets from chicken; discard or save for another use. Rinse chicken body cavity; pat dry with paper towels. Snip any excess skin or fat from chicken.

2. In a food processor combine olive oil, garlic, lemon peel, thyme, pepper, and saffron. Process to form a smooth paste.

3. Using fingers, rub paste over the outside surface of the chicken and the inside cavity. Transfer chicken to a large bowl; cover and refrigerate for at least 8 hours or overnight.

4. Preheat oven to 425°F. Place lemon quarters and bay leaves in chicken cavity. Tie legs together with 100%-cotton kitchen string. Tuck wings under chicken. Insert an oven-going meat thermometer into the inside thigh muscle without touching bone. Place chicken on a rack in a large roasting pan.

5. Roast for 15 minutes. Reduce oven temperature to 375°F. Roast about 1 hour more or until juices run clear and thermometer registers 175°F. Tent chicken with foil. Let stand for 10 minutes before carving.

SPATCHCOCKED CHICKEN WITH JICAMA SLAW

PREP: 40 minutes GRILL: 1 hour 5 minutes STAND: 10 minutes MAKES: 4 servings

"SPATCHCOCK" IS AN OLD COOKING TERM THAT'S RECENTLY COME BACK INTO USE TO DESCRIBE THE PROCESS OF SPLITTING A SMALL BIRD—SUCH AS A CHICKEN OR CORNISH HEN—DOWN THE BACK AND THEN OPENING IT AND FLATTENING IT LIKE A BOOK TO HELP IT COOK QUICKLY AND MORE EVENLY. IT'S SIMILAR TO BUTTERFLYING BUT REFERS ONLY TO POULTRY.

CHICKEN

- 1 poblano chile
- 1 tablespoon finely chopped shallot
- 3 cloves garlic, minced
- 1 teaspoon finely shredded lemon peel
- 1 teaspoon finely shredded lime peel
- 1 teaspoon Smoky Seasoning (see recipe)
- ½ teaspoon dried oregano, crushed
- ½ teaspoon ground cumin
- 1 tablespoon olive oil
- 1 3- to 3½–pound whole chicken

SLAW

- ½ of a medium jicama, peeled and cut into julienne strips (about 3 cups)
- ½ cup thinly sliced scallions (4)
- 1 Granny Smith apple, peeled, cored, and cut into julienne strips
- ⅓ cup snipped fresh cilantro
- 3 tablespoons fresh orange juice
- 3 tablespoons olive oil
- 1 teaspoon Lemon-Herb Seasoning (see recipe)

1. For a charcoal grill, arrange medium hot coals on one side of the grill. Place a drip pan under the empty side of the grill. Place poblano on the grill rack directly over medium coals. Cover and grill for 15 minutes or until the poblano is charred on all sides, turning occasionally. Immediately wrap poblano in foil; let stand for 10 minutes. Open foil and cut poblano in half lengthwise; remove stems and seeds (see tip). Using a sharp knife, gently peel off skin and discard. Finely chop the poblano. (For a gas grill, preheat grill; reduce heat to medium. Adjust for indirect cooking. Grill as above over burner that is turned on.)

2. For the rub, in a small bowl combine poblano, shallot, garlic, lemon peel, lime peel, Smoky Seasoning, oregano, and cumin. Stir in oil; mix well to make a paste.

3. To spatchcock the chicken, remove the neck and giblets from chicken (save for another use). Place the chicken, breast side down, on a cutting board. Use kitchen shears to make a lengthwise cut down one side of the backbone, starting from the neck end. Repeat the lengthwise cut to opposite side of the backbone. Remove and discard the backbone. Turn chicken skin side up. Press down between the breasts to break the breast bone so the chicken lies flat.

4. Starting at the neck on one side of the breast, slip your fingers between skin and meat, loosening skin as you work toward the thigh. Free the skin around the thigh.

Repeat on the other side. Use your fingers to spread rub over the meat under the skin of the chicken.

5. Place chicken, breast side down, on grill rack over drip pan. Weight with two foil-wrapped bricks or a large cast-iron skillet. Cover and grill for 30 minutes. Turn chicken, bone side down, on rack, weighting again with bricks or skillet. Grill, covered, about 30 minutes more or until chicken is no longer pink (175°F in thigh muscle). Remove chicken from grill; let stand for 10 minutes. (For a gas grill, place chicken on grill rack away from heat. Grill as above.)

6. Meanwhile, for the slaw, in a large bowl combine jicama, scallions, apple, and cilantro. In a small bowl whisk together orange juice, oil, and Lemon-Herb Seasoning. Pour over the jicama mixture and toss to coat. Serve chicken with the slaw.

ROASTED CHICKEN HINDQUARTERS WITH VODKA, CARROT, AND TOMATO SAUCE

PREP: 15 minutes COOK: 15 minutes ROAST: 30 minutes MAKES: 4 servings

VODKA CAN BE MADE FROM SEVERAL DIFFERENT FOODSTUFFS, INCLUDING POTATOES, CORN, RYE, WHEAT, AND BARLEY—EVEN GRAPES. ALTHOUGH THERE ISN'T MUCH VODKA IN THIS SAUCE WHEN YOU DIVIDE IT AMONG FOUR SERVINGS, LOOK FOR VOKDA MADE FROM EITHER POTATOES OR GRAPES TO BE PALEO COMPLIANT.

3 tablespoons olive oil

4 bone-in chicken hindquarters or meaty chicken pieces, skinned

1 28-ounce can no-salt-added plum tomatoes, drained

½ cup finely chopped onion

½ cup finely chopped carrot

3 cloves garlic, minced

1 teaspoon Mediterranean Seasoning (see recipe)

⅛ teaspoon cayenne pepper

1 sprig fresh rosemary

2 tablespoons vodka

1 tablespoon snipped fresh basil (optional)

1. Preheat oven to 375°F. In an extra-large skillet heat 2 tablespoons of the oil over medium-high heat. Add chicken; cook about 12 minutes or until browned, turning to brown evenly. Place skillet in the preheated oven. Roast, uncovered, for 20 minutes.

2. Meanwhile, for sauce, use kitchen scissors to cut up the tomatoes. In a medium saucepan heat the remaining 1 tablespoon oil over medium heat. Add onion, carrot, and garlic; cook for 3 minutes or until tender, stirring frequently. Stir in snipped tomatoes, Mediterranean Seasoning, cayenne pepper, and rosemary sprig. Bring to boiling over medium-high heat; reduce heat. Simmer, uncovered, for 10 minutes, stirring occasionally. Stir in vodka; cook 1 minute more; remove and discard rosemary sprig.

3. Ladle sauce over chicken in skillet. Return skillet to oven. Roast, covered, about 10 minutes more or until chicken is tender and no longer pink (175°F). If desired, sprinkle with basil.

POULET RÔTI AND RUTABAGA FRITES

PREP: 40 minutes BAKE: 40 minutes MAKES: 4 servings

THE CRISP RUTABAGA FRITES ARE DELICIOUS SERVED WITH THE ROASTED CHICKEN AND ITS ATTENDANT COOKING JUICES—BUT THEY ARE EQUALLY TASTY MADE ON THEIR OWN AND SERVED WITH PALEO KETCHUP (SEE RECIPE) OR SERVED BELGIAN-STYLE WITH PALEO AÏOLI (GARLIC MAYO, SEE RECIPE).

6 tablespoons olive oil

1 tablespoon Mediterranean Seasoning (see recipe)

4 bone-in chicken thighs, skinned (about 1 ¼ pounds total)

4 chicken drumsticks, skinned (about 1 pound total)

1 cup dry white wine

1 cup Chicken Bone Broth (see recipe) or no-salt-added chicken broth

1 small onion, quartered

Olive oil

1½ to 2 pounds rutabagas

2 tablespoons snipped fresh chives

Black pepper

1. Preheat oven to 400°F. In a small bowl combine 1 tablespoon of the olive oil and the Mediterranean Seasoning; rub onto chicken pieces. In an extra-large oven-going skillet heat 2 tablespoons of the oil. Add chicken pieces, meaty sides down. Cook, uncovered, about 5 minutes or until browned. Remove skillet from heat. Turn chicken pieces, browned sides up. Add wine, Chicken Bone Broth, and onion.

2. Place skillet in oven on middle rack. Bake, uncovered, for 10 minutes.

3. Meanwhile, for frites, lightly brush a large baking sheet with olive oil; set aside. Peel rutabagas. Using a sharp knife, cut rutabagas into ½-inch slices. Cut slices lengthwise into ½-inch strips. In a large bowl toss rutabaga strips with the remaining 3 tablespoons oil. Spread rutabaga strips in a single layer on prepared baking sheet; place in oven on top rack. Bake for 15 minutes; turn frites over. Bake chicken for 10 minutes more or until no longer pink (175°F). Remove chicken from oven. Bake frites 5 to 10 minutes or until browned and tender.

4. Remove chicken and onion from skillet, reserving juices. Cover chicken and onion to keep warm. Bring juices to boiling over medium heat; reduce heat. Simmer, uncovered, about 5 minutes more or until juices are slightly reduced.

5. To serve, toss frites with chives and season with pepper. Serve chicken with cooking juices and frites.

TRIPLE-MUSHROOM COQ AU VIN WITH CHIVE MASHED RUTABAGAS

PREP: 15 minutes COOK: 1 hour 15 minutes MAKES: 4 to 6 servings

IF THERE IS ANY GRIT IN THE BOWL AFTER SOAKING THE DRIED MUSHROOMS—AND IT IS LIKELY THAT THERE WILL BE—STRAIN THE LIQUID THROUGH A DOUBLE THICKNESS OF CHEESECLOTH SET IN A FINE-MESH STRAINER.

1 ounce dried porcini or morel mushrooms

1 cup boiling water

2 to 2½ pounds chicken thighs and drumsticks, skinned

Black pepper

2 tablespoons olive oil

2 medium leeks, halved lengthwise, rinsed, and thinly sliced

2 portobello mushrooms, sliced

8 ounces fresh oyster mushrooms, stemmed and sliced, or sliced fresh button mushrooms

¼ cup no-salt-added tomato paste

1 teaspoon dried marjoram, crushed

½ teaspoon dried thyme, crushed

½ cup dry red wine

6 cups Chicken Bone Broth (see recipe) or no-salt-added chicken broth

2 bay leaves

2 to 2½ pounds rutabagas, peeled and chopped

2 tablespoons snipped fresh chives

½ teaspoon black pepper

Snipped fresh thyme (optional)

1. In a small bowl combine the porcini mushrooms and the boiling water; let stand for 15 minutes. Remove mushrooms, reserving the soaking liquid. Chop the

mushrooms. Set the mushrooms and soaking liquid aside.

2. Sprinkle chicken with pepper. In an extra-large skillet with a tight-fitting lid heat 1 tablespoon of the olive oil over medium-high heat. Cook chicken pieces, in two batches, in hot oil about 15 minutes until lightly browned, turning once. Remove chicken from the skillet. Stir in leeks, portobello mushrooms, and oyster mushrooms. Cook for 4 to 5 minutes or just until mushrooms start to brown, stirring occasionally. Stir in tomato paste, marjoram, and thyme; cook and stir for 1 minute. Stir in wine; cook and stir for 1 minute. Stir in 3 cups of the Chicken Bone Broth, bay leaves, ½ cup of the reserved mushroom soaking liquid, and rehydrated chopped mushrooms. Return chicken to skillet. Bring to boiling; reduce heat. Simmer, covered, about 45 minutes or until chicken is tender, turning the chicken once halfway through cooking.

3. Meanwhile, in a large saucepan combine rutabagas and the remaining 3 cups broth. If necessary, add water to just cover rutabagas. Bring to boiling; reduce heat. Simmer, uncovered, for 25 to 30 minutes or until rutabagas are tender, stirring occasionally. Drain rutabagas, reserving liquid. Return rutabagas to the saucepan. Add the remaining 1 tablespoon olive oil, the chives, and the ½ teaspoon pepper. Using a potato masher, mash the rutabaga mixture, adding cooking liquid as needed to make desired consistency.

4. Remove bay leaves from chicken mixture; discard. Serve chicken and sauce over mashed rutabagas. If desired, sprinkle with fresh thyme.

PEACH-BRANDY-GLAZED DRUMSTICKS

PREP: 30 minutes GRILL: 40 minutes MAKES: 4 servings

THESE CHICKEN LEGS ARE PERFECT WITH A CRISPY SLAW AND THE SPICY OVEN-BAKED SWEET POTATO FRIES FROM THE RECIPE FOR TUNISIAN SPICE-RUBBED PORK SHOULDER (SEE RECIPE). THEY'RE SHOWN HERE WITH CRUNCHY CABBAGE SLAW WITH RADISHES, MANGO, AND MINT (SEE RECIPE).

PEACH-BRANDY GLAZE

1 tablespoon olive oil

½ cup chopped onion

2 fresh medium peaches, halved, pitted, and chopped

2 tablespoons brandy

1 cup BBQ Sauce (see recipe)

8 chicken drumsticks (2 to 2½ pounds total), skinned if desired

1. For glaze, in a medium saucepan heat olive oil over medium heat. Add onion; cook about 5 minutes or until tender, stirring occasionally. Add peaches. Cover and cook for 4 to 6 minutes or until peaches are tender, stirring occasionally. Add brandy; cook, uncovered, for 2 minutes, stirring occasionally. Cool slightly. Transfer peach mixture to a blender or food processor. Cover and blend or process until smooth. Add BBQ Sauce. Cover and blend or process until smooth. Return sauce to the saucepan. Cook over medium-low heat just until heated through. Transfer ¾ cup of the sauce to a small

bowl for brushing on the chicken. Keep remaining sauce warm for serving with grilled chicken.

2. For a charcoal grill, arrange medium-hot coals around a drip pan. Test for medium heat above drip pan. Place chicken drumsticks on grill rack over drip pan. Cover and grill for 40 to 50 minutes or until chicken is no longer pink (175°F), turning once halfway through grilling and brushing with ¾ cup of the Peach-Brandy Glaze for the last 5 to 10 minutes of grilling. (For a gas grill, preheat grill. Reduce heat to medium. Adjust heat for indirect cooking. Add chicken drumsticks to grill rack that is not over the heat. Cover and grill as directed.)

CHILE-MARINATED CHICKEN WITH MANGO-MELON SALAD

PREP: 40 minutes CHILL/MARINATE: 2 to 4 hours GRILL: 50 minutes MAKES: 6 to 8 servings

AN ANCHO CHILE IS A DRIED POBLANO—A GLOSSY, DEEP-GREEN CHILE WITH AN INTENSELY FRESH FLAVOR. ANCHO CHILES HAVE A SLIGHTLY FRUITY FLAVOR WITH A HINT OF PLUM OR RAISIN AND JUST A TOUCH OF BITTERNESS. NEW MEXICO CHILES CAN BE MODERATELY HOT. THEY'RE THE DEEP-RED CHILES YOU SEE BUNCHED AND HANGING IN RISTRAS—COLORFUL ARRANGEMENTS OF DRYING CHILES—IN PARTS OF THE SOUTHWEST.

CHICKEN

- 2 dried New Mexico chiles
- 2 dried ancho chiles
- 1 cup boiling water
- 3 tablespoons olive oil
- 1 large sweet onion, peeled and cut into thick slices
- 4 roma tomatoes, cored
- 1 tablespoon minced garlic (6 cloves)
- 2 teaspoons ground cumin
- 1 teaspoon dried oregano, crushed
- 16 chicken drumsticks

SALAD

- 2 cups cubed cantaloupe
- 2 cups cubed honeydew
- 2 cups cubed mango
- ¼ cup fresh lime juice
- 1 teaspoon chili powder

59

½ teaspoon ground cumin

¼ cup snipped fresh cilantro

1. For chicken, remove stems and seeds from dried New Mexico and ancho chiles. Heat a large skillet over medium heat. Toast chiles in the skillet for 1 to 2 minutes or until fragrant and lightly toasted. Place toasted chiles in a small bowl; add the boiling water to the bowl. Let stand at least 10 minutes or until ready to use.

2. Preheat the broiler. Line a baking sheet with foil; brush 1 tablespoon of the olive oil over foil. Place onion slices and tomatoes on pan. Broil about 4 inches from heat for 6 to 8 minutes or until softened and charred. Drain chiles, reserving the water.

3. For marinade, in a blender or food processor combine chiles, onion, tomatoes, garlic, cumin, and oregano. Cover and blend or process until smooth, adding reserved water as needed to puree and reach desired consistency.

4. Place chicken in a large resealable plastic bag set in a shallow dish. Pour marinade over chicken in bag, turning bag to coat evenly. Marinate in refrigerator for 2 to 4 hours, turning bag occasionally.

5. For salad, in an extra-large bowl combine cantaloupe, honeydew, mango, lime juice, the remaining 2 tablespoons olive oil, chili powder, cumin, and cilantro. Toss to coat. Cover and chill for 1 to 4 hours.

6. For a charcoal grill, arrange medium-hot coals around a drip pan. Test for medium heat above the pan. Drain

chicken, reserving the marinade. Place chicken on the grill rack over the drip pan. Brush chicken generously with some of the reserved marinade (discard any extra marinade). Cover and grill for 50 minutes or until chicken is no longer pink (175°F), turning once halfway through grilling. (For a gas grill, preheat grill. Reduce heat to medium. Adjust for indirect cooking. Continue as directed, placing chicken on the burner that is turned off.) Serve chicken drumsticks with salad.

TANDOORI-STYLE CHICKEN LEGS WITH CUCUMBER RAITA

PREP: 20 minutes MARINATE: 2 to 24 hours BROIL: 25 minutes MAKES: 4 servings

THE RAITA IS MADE WITH CASHEW CREAM, LEMON JUICE, MINT, CILANTRO, AND CUCUMBER. IT PROVIDES A COOLING COUNTERPOINT TO THE HOT AND SPICY CHICKEN.

CHICKEN

- 1 onion, cut into thin wedges
- 1 2-inch piece fresh ginger, peeled and quartered
- 4 cloves garlic
- 3 tablespoons olive oil
- 2 tablespoons fresh lemon juice
- 1 teaspoon ground cumin
- 1 teaspoon ground turmeric
- ½ teaspoon ground allspice
- ½ teaspoon ground cinnamon
- ½ teaspoon black pepper
- ¼ teaspoon cayenne pepper
- 8 chicken drumsticks

CUCUMBER RAITA

- 1 cup Cashew Cream (see recipe)
- 1 tablespoon fresh lemon juice
- 1 tablespoon snipped fresh mint
- 1 tablespoon snipped fresh cilantro
- ½ teaspoon ground cumin
- ⅛ teaspoon black pepper
- 1 medium cucumber, peeled, seeded, and diced (1 cup)
- Lemon wedges

1. In a blender or food processor combine onion, ginger, garlic, olive oil, lemon juice, cumin, turmeric, allspice, cinnamon, black pepper, and cayenne pepper. Cover and blend or process until smooth.

2. Using the tip of a paring knife, pierce each drumstick four or five times. Place drumsticks in a large resealable plastic bag set in a large bowl. Add onion mixture; turn to coat. Marinate in the refrigerator for 2 to 24 hours, turning bag occasionally.

3. Preheat broiler. Remove chicken from marinade. Using paper towels, wipe excess marinade from drumsticks. Arrange drumsticks on the rack of an unheated broiler pan or rimmed baking sheet lined with foil. Broil 6 to 8 inches from heat source for 15 minutes. Turn drumsticks over; broil about 10 minutes or until chicken is no longer pink (175°F).

4. For the raita, in a medium bowl combine Cashew Cream, lemon juice, mint, cilantro, cumin, and black pepper. Gently stir in cucumber.

5. Serve chicken with raita and lemon wedges.

CURRIED CHICKEN STEW WITH ROOT VEGETABLES, ASPARAGUS, AND GREEN APPLE-MINT RELISH

PREP: 30 minutes COOK: 35 minutes STAND: 5 minutes MAKES: 4 servings

2 tablespoons refined coconut oil or olive oil

2 pounds bone-in chicken breasts, skinned if desired

1 cup chopped onion

2 tablespoons grated fresh ginger

2 tablespoons minced garlic

2 tablespoons salt-free curry powder

2 tablespoons minced, seeded jalapeño (see tip)

4 cups Chicken Bone Broth (see recipe) or no-salt-added chicken broth

2 medium sweet potatoes (about 1 pound), peeled and chopped

2 medium turnips (about 6 ounces), peeled and chopped

1 cup seeded, diced tomato

8 ounces asparagus, trimmed and cut into 1-inch lengths

1 13.5-ounce can natural coconut milk (such as Nature's Way)

½ cup snipped fresh cilantro

Apple-Mint Relish (see recipe, below)

Lime wedges

1. In a 6-quart Dutch oven heat oil over medium-high heat. Brown chicken in batches in hot oil, turning to brown evenly, about 10 minutes. Transfer chicken to a plate; set aside.

2. Turn heat to medium. Add onion, ginger, garlic, curry powder, and jalapeño to the pot. Cook and stir 5 minutes or until onion is softened. Stir in Chicken Bone Broth, sweet potatoes, turnips, and tomato. Return the chicken pieces to the pot, arranging to submerge chicken in as much liquid as possible. Reduce heat to

64

medium-low. Cover and simmer 30 minutes or until chicken is no longer pink and vegetables are tender. Stir in asparagus, coconut milk, and cilantro. Remove from heat. Let stand for 5 minutes. Cut chicken from bones, if necessary, to divide evenly among serving bowls. Serve with Apple-Mint Relish and lime wedges.

Apple-Mint Relish: In a food processor chop ½ cup unsweetened coconut flakes until powdery. Add 1 cup fresh cilantro leaves and steams; 1 cup fresh mint leaves; 1 Granny Smith apple, cored and chopped; 2 teaspoons minced, seeded jalapeño (see tip); and 1 tablespoon fresh lime juice. Pulse until finely minced.

GRILLED CHICKEN PAILLARD SALAD WITH RASPBERRIES, BEETS, AND ROASTED ALMONDS

PREP: 30 minutes ROAST: 45 minutes MARINATE: 15 minutes GRILL: 8 minutes
MAKES: 4 servings

½ cup whole almonds

1½ teaspoons olive oil

1 medium red beet

1 medium golden beet

2 6- to 8-ounce boneless, skinless chicken breast halves

2 cups fresh or frozen raspberries, thawed

3 tablespoons white or red wine vinegar

2 tablespoons snipped fresh tarragon

1 tablespoon minced shallot

1 teaspoon Dijon-Style Mustard (see recipe)

¼ cup olive oil

 Black pepper

8 cups spring mix lettuces

1. For the almonds, preheat the oven to 400°F. Spread almonds on a small baking sheet and toss with ½ teaspoon olive oil. Bake about 5 minutes or until fragrant and golden. Let cool. (Almonds may be toasted 2 days ahead and stored in an airtight container.)

2. For the beets, place each beet on a small piece of foil and drizzle with each with ½ teaspoon olive oil. Loosely wrap the foil around the beets and place on a baking sheet or in a baking dish. Roast the beets in the 400°F oven for 40 to 50 minutes or until tender when pierced with a knife. Remove from oven and let stand until cool enough to handle. Using a paring knife, remove the

skin. Cut beets into wedges and set aside. (Avoid mixing the beets together to prevent the red beets from staining the golden beets. Beets may be roasted 1 day ahead and chilled. Bring to room temperature before serving.)

3. For the chicken, cut each chicken breast in half horizontally. Place each piece of chicken between two pieces of plastic wrap. Using a meat mallet, gently pound to about ¾ inch thick. Place chicken in a shallow dish and set aside.

4. For vinaigrette, in a large bowl lightly crush ¾ cup of the raspberries with a whisk (reserve remaining raspberries for the salad). Add the vinegar, tarragon, shallot, and Dijon-Style Mustard; whisk to blend. Add the ¼ cup olive oil in a thin stream, whisking to mix well. Pour ½ cup vinaigrette over the chicken; turn chicken to coat (reserve remaining vinaigrette for the salad). Marinate chicken at room temperature for 15 minutes. Remove chicken from the marinade and sprinkle with pepper; discard marinade remaining in dish.

5. For a charcoal or gas grill, place chicken on a grill rack directly over medium heat. Cover and grill for 8 to 10 minutes or until chicken is no longer pink, turning once halfway through grilling. (Chicken can also be cooked in a stovetop grill pan.)

6. In a large bowl combine lettuce, beets, and the remaining 1¼ cups raspberries. Pour reserved vinaigrette over salad; gently toss to coat. Divide salad among four serving plates; top each with a grilled chicken breast

piece. Coarsely chop the roasted almonds and sprinkle over all. Serve immediately.

BROCCOLI RABE-STUFFED CHICKEN BREASTS WITH FRESH TOMATO SAUCE AND CAESAR SALAD

PREP: 40 minutes COOK: 25 minutes MAKES: 6 servings

3 tablespoons olive oil

2 teaspoons minced garlic

¼ teaspoon crushed red pepper

1 pound broccoli raab, trimmed and chopped

½ cup unsulfured golden raisins

½ cup water

4 5- to 6-ounce skinless, boneless chicken breast halves

1 cup chopped onion

3 cups chopped tomatoes

¼ cup snipped fresh basil

2 teaspoons red wine vinegar

3 tablespoons fresh lemon juice

2 tablespoons Paleo Mayo (see recipe)

2 teaspoons Dijon-Style Mustard (see recipe)

1 teaspoon minced garlic

½ teaspoon black pepper

¼ cup olive oil

10 cups chopped romaine lettuce

1. In a large skillet heat 1 tablespoon of the olive oil over medium-high heat. Add the garlic and crushed red pepper; cook and stir for 30 seconds or until fragrant. Add the chopped broccoli rabe, raisins, and the ½ cup water. Cover and cook about 8 minutes or until broccoli raab is wilted and tender. Remove lid from pan; let any excess water evaporate. Set aside.

2. For roulades, halve each chicken breast lengthwise; place each piece between two pieces of plastic wrap. Using the flat side of a meat mallet, pound chicken lightly to about ¼ inch thick. For each roulade, place about ¼ cup of the broccoli raab mixture on one of the short ends; roll up, folding in the sides to completely enclose filling. (Roulades may be made up to 1 day ahead and chilled until ready to cook.)

3. In a large skillet heat 1 tablespoon of the olive oil over medium-high heat. Add the roulades, seam sides down. Cook about 8 minutes or until browned on all sides, turning two or three times during cooking. Transfer roulades to a platter.

4. For sauce, in the skillet heat 1 tablespoon of the remaining olive oil over medium heat. Add the onion; cook about 5 minutes or until translucent. Stir in the tomatoes and basil. Place roulades on top of the sauce in skillet. Bring to boiling over medium-high heat; reduce heat. Cover and simmer about 5 minutes or until tomatoes start to break down but still retain their shape and roulades are heated through.

5. For dressing, in a small bowl whisk together the lemon juice, Paleo Mayo, Dijon-Style Mustard, garlic, and black pepper. Drizzle in the ¼ cup olive oil, whisking until emulsified. In a large bowl toss dressing with the chopped romaine. To serve, divide romaine among six serving plates. Slice roulades and arrange on romaine; drizzle with tomato sauce.

GRILLED CHICKEN SHAWARMA WRAPS WITH SPICED VEGETABLES AND PINE NUT DRESSING

PREP: 20 minutes MARINATE: 30 minutes GRILL: 10 minutes MAKES: 8 wraps (4 servings)

1½ pounds skinless, boneless chicken breast halves, cut into 2-inch pieces

5 tablespoons olive oil

2 tablespoons fresh lemon juice

1¾ teaspoons ground cumin

1 teaspoon minced garlic

1 teaspoon paprika

½ teaspoon curry powder

½ teaspoon ground cinnamon

¼ teaspoon cayenne pepper

1 medium zucchini, halved

1 small eggplant cut into ½-inch slices

1 large yellow sweet pepper, halved and seeded

1 medium red onion, quartered

8 cherry tomatoes

8 large butter lettuce leaves

Toasted Pine Nut Dressing (see recipe)

Lemon wedges

1. For marinade, in a small bowl combine 3 tablespoons of the olive oil, lemon juice, 1 teaspoon of the cumin, garlic, ½ teaspoon of the paprika, curry powder, ¼ teaspoon of the cinnamon, and cayenne pepper. Place chicken pieces in a large resealable plastic bag set in a shallow dish. Pour marinade over the chicken. Seal bag;

turn bag to coat. Marinate in the refrigerator for 30 minutes, turning bag occasionally.

2. Remove chicken from marinade; discard marinade. Thread chicken on four long skewers.

3. Place zucchini, eggplant, sweet pepper, and onion on a baking sheet. Drizzle with 2 tablespoons of the olive oil. Sprinkle with the remaining ¾ teaspoon cumin, remaining ½ teaspoon paprika, and the remaining ¼ teaspoon cinnamon; lightly rub over vegetables. Thread tomatoes on two skewers.

3. For a charcoal or gas grill, place chicken and tomato kabobs and vegetables on a grill rack over medium heat. Cover and grill until chicken is no longer pink and vegetables are lightly charred and crisp-tender, turning once. Allow 10 to 12 minutes for chicken, 8 to 10 minutes for vegetables, and 4 minutes for tomatoes.

4. Remove chicken from skewers. Chop chicken and cut zucchini, eggplant, and sweet pepper into bite-size pieces. Remove the tomatoes from skewers (do not chop). Arrange chicken and vegetables on a platter. To serve, spoon some of the chicken and vegetables into a lettuce leaf; drizzle with Toasted Pine Nut Dressing. Serve with lemon wedges.

OVEN-BRAISED CHICKEN BREASTS WITH MUSHROOMS, GARLIC-MASHED CAULIFLOWER, AND ROASTED ASPARAGUS

START TO FINISH: 50 minutes MAKES: 4 servings

4 10- to 12-ounce bone-in chicken breast halves, skinned

3 cups small white button mushrooms

1 cup thinly sliced leeks or yellow onion

2 cups Chicken Bone Broth (see recipe) or no-salt-added chicken broth

1 cup dry white wine

1 large bunch fresh thyme

Black pepper

White wine vinegar (optional)

1 head cauliflower, separated into florets

12 cloves garlic, peeled

2 tablespoons olive oil

White or cayenne pepper

1 pound asparagus, trimmed

2 teaspoons olive oil

1. Preheat oven to 400°F. Arrange chicken breasts in a 3-quart rectangular baking dish; top with mushrooms and leeks. Pour Chicken Bone Broth and wine over the chicken and vegetables. Scatter thyme over all and sprinkle with black pepper. Cover dish with foil.

2. Bake for 35 to 40 minutes or until an instant-read thermometer inserted in chicken registers 170°F. Remove and discard thyme sprigs. If desired, season braising liquid with a splash of vinegar before serving.

2. Meanwhile, in a large saucepan cook cauliflower and garlic in enough boiling water to cover about 10 minutes or until very tender. Drain cauliflower and garlic, reserving 2 tablespoons of the cooking liquid. In a food processor or a large mixing bowl place cauliflower and reserved cooking liquid. Process until smooth* or mash with a potato masher; stir in 2 tablespoons olive oil and season to taste with white pepper. Keep warm until ready to serve.

3. Arrange asparagus in a single layer on a baking sheet. Drizzle with 2 teaspoons olive oil and toss to coat. Sprinkle with black pepper. Roast in a 400°F oven about 8 minutes or until crisp-tender, stirring once.

4. Divide mashed cauliflower among six serving plates. Top with chicken, mushrooms, and leeks. Drizzle with some of the braising liquid; serve with roasted asparagus.

*Note: If using a food processor, be careful not to overprocess or cauliflower will get too thin.

THAI-STYLE CHICKEN SOUP

PREP: 30 minutes FREEZE: 20 minutes COOK: 50 minutes MAKES: 4 to 6 servings

TAMARIND IS A MUSKY, SOUR FRUIT USED IN INDIAN, THAI, AND MEXICAN COOKING. MANY COMMERCIALLY PREPARED TAMARIND PASTES CONTAIN SUGAR—BE SURE YOU PURCHASE ONE THAT DOES NOT. KAFFIR LIME LEAVES CAN BE FOUND FRESH, FROZEN, AND DRIED AT MOST ASIAN MARKETS. IF YOU CAN'T FIND THEM, SUBSTITUTE 1½ TEASPOONS FINELY SHREDDED LIME PEEL FOR THE LEAVES IN THIS RECIPE.

2 stalks lemongrass, trimmed

2 tablespoons unrefined coconut oil

½ cup thinly sliced scallions

3 large cloves garlic, thinly sliced

8 cups Chicken Bone Broth (see recipe) or no-salt-added chicken broth

¼ cup no-sugar-added tamarind paste (such as Tamicon brand)

2 tablespoons nori flakes

3 fresh Thai chiles, thinly sliced with seeds intact (see tip)

3 kaffir lime leaves

1 3-inch piece ginger, thinly sliced

4 6-ounce skinless, boneless chicken breast halves

1 14.5-ounce can no-salt-added fire-roasted diced tomatoes, undrained

6 ounces thin asparagus spears, trimmed and thinly sliced diagonally into ½-inch pieces

½ cup packed Thai basil leaves (see note)

1. Using the back of a knife with firm pressure, bruise the lemongrass stalks. Finely chop bruised stalks.

2. In a Dutch oven heat coconut oil over medium heat. Add lemongrass and scallions; cook for 8 to 10 minutes,

stirring often. Add garlic; cook and stir for 2 to 3 minutes or until very fragrant.

3. Add Chicken Bone Broth, tamarind paste, nori flakes, chiles, lime leaves, and ginger. Bring to boiling; reduce heat. Cover and simmer for 40 minutes.

4. Meanwhile, freeze chicken for 20 to 30 minutes or until firm. Thinly slice chicken.

5. Strain soup through a fine-mesh sieve into a large saucepan, pressing with the back of a large spoon to extract flavors. Discard solids. Bring soup to boiling. Stir in chicken, undrained tomatoes, asparagus, and basil. Reduce heat; simmer, uncovered, for 2 to 3 minutes or until chicken is cooked through. Serve immediately.

LEMON AND SAGE ROASTED CHICKEN WITH ENDIVE

PREP: 15 minutes ROAST: 55 minutes STAND: 5 minutes MAKES: 4 servings

THE LEMON SLICES AND SAGE LEAF PLACED UNDER THE SKIN OF THE CHICKEN FLAVOR THE MEAT AS IT COOKS— AND MAKE AN EYE-CATCHING DESIGN UNDER THE CRISP, OPAQUE SKIN AFTER IT COMES OUT OF THE OVEN.

- 4 bone-in chicken breast halves (with skin)
- 1 lemon, very thinly sliced
- 4 large sage leaves
- 2 teaspoons olive oil
- 2 teaspoons Mediterranean Seasoning (see recipe)
- ½ teaspoon black pepper
- 2 tablespoons extra virgin olive oil
- 2 shallots, sliced
- 2 cloves garlic, minced
- 4 heads endive, halved lengthwise

1. Preheat oven to 400°F. Using a paring knife, very carefully loosen the skin from each breast half, leaving it attached on one side. Place 2 lemon slices and 1 sage leaf on the meat of each breast. Gently pull skin back into place and press gently to secure it.

2. Arrange chicken in a shallow roasting pan. Brush chicken with 2 teaspoons olive oil; sprinkle with Mediterranean Seasoning and ¼ teaspoon of the pepper. Roast, uncovered, about 55 minutes or until skin is browned and crisp and an instant-read thermometer inserted into

77

chicken registers 170°F. Let chicken stand for 10 minutes before serving.

3. Meanwhile, in a large skillet heat the 2 tablespoons olive oil over medium heat. Add shallots; cook about 2 minutes or until translucent. Sprinkle endive with the remaining ¼ teaspoon pepper. Add garlic to skillet. Place endive in skillet, cut sides down. Cook about 5 minutes or until browned. Carefully turn endive over; cook for 2 to 3 minutes more or until tender. Serve with chicken.

CHICKEN WITH SCALLIONS, WATERCRESS, AND RADISHES

PREP: 20 minutes COOK: 8 minutes BAKE: 30 minutes MAKES: 4 servings

ALTHOUGH IT MIGHT SOUND ODD TO COOK RADISHES, THEY ARE BARELY COOKED HERE—JUST ENOUGH TO MELLOW THEIR PEPPERY BITE AND TENDERIZE THEM A BIT.

3 tablespoons olive oil

4 10- to 12-ounce bone-in chicken breast halves (with skin)

1 tablespoon Lemon-Herb Seasoning (see recipe)

¾ cup sliced scallions

6 radishes, thinly sliced

¼ teaspoon black pepper

½ cup dry white vermouth or dry white wine

⅓ cup Cashew Cream (see recipe)

1 bunch watercress, stems trimmed, roughly chopped

1 tablespoon snipped fresh dill

1. Preheat oven to 350°F. In a large skillet heat olive oil over medium-high heat. Pat chicken dry with a paper towel. Cook chicken, skin sides down, for 4 to 5 minutes or until skin is golden and crisp. Turn chicken over; cook about 4 minutes or until browned. Arrange chicken, skin sides up, in a shallow baking dish. Sprinkle chicken with Lemon-Herb Seasoning. Bake about 30 minutes or until an instant-read thermometer inserted into chicken registers 170°F.

2. Meanwhile, pour all but 1 tablespoon drippings from skillet; return skillet to heat. Add scallions and radishes;

cook about 3 minutes or just until scallions wilt. Sprinkle with pepper. Add vermouth, stirring to scrape up browned bits. Bring to boiling; cook until reduced and slightly thickened. Stir in Cashew Cream; bring to boiling. Remove skillet from heat; add watercress and dill, stirring gently just until watercress wilts. Stir in any chicken juices that have accumulated in the baking dish.

3. Divide scallion mixture among four serving plates; top with chicken.

CHICKEN TIKKA MASALA

PREP: 30 minutes MARINATE: 4 to 6 hours COOK: 15 minutes BROIL: 8 minutes
MAKES: 4 servings

THIS WAS INSPIRED BY A VERY POPULAR INDIAN DISH THAT MAY NOT HAVE BEEN CREATED IN INDIA AT ALL, BUT RATHER AT AN INDIAN RESTAURANT IN THE UNITED KINGDOM. TRADITIONAL CHICKEN TIKKA MASALA CALLS FOR CHICKEN TO BE MARINATED IN YOGURT AND THEN COOKED IN A SPICY TOMATO SAUCE SPLASHED WITH CREAM. WITHOUT ANY DAIRY BLUNTING THE FLAVOR OF THE SAUCE, THIS VERSION IS ESPECIALLY CLEAN-TASTING. INSTEAD OF RICE, IT'S SERVED OVER CRISP ZUCCHINI NOODLES.

1½ pounds skinless, boneless chicken thighs or chicken breast halves

¾ cup natural coconut milk (such as Nature's Way)

6 cloves garlic, minced

1 tablespoon grated fresh ginger

1 teaspoon ground coriander

1 teaspoon paprika

1 teaspoon ground cumin

¼ teaspoon ground cardamom

4 tablespoons refined coconut oil

1 cup chopped carrots

1 thinly sliced celery

½ cup chopped onion

2 jalapeño or serrano chiles, seeded (if desired) and finely chopped (see tip)

1 14.5-ounce can no-salt-added fire-roasted diced tomatoes, undrained

1 8-ounce can no-salt-added tomato sauce

1 teaspoon no-salt-added garam masala

3 medium zucchini

½ teaspoon black pepper

81

Fresh cilantro leaves

1. If using chicken thighs, cut each thigh into three pieces. If using chicken breast halves, cut each breast half into 2-inch pieces, cutting any thick portions in half horizontally to make them thinner. Place chicken in a large resealable plastic bag; set aside. For marinade, in a small bowl combine ½ cup of the coconut milk, the garlic, ginger, coriander, paprika, cumin, and cardamom. Pour marinade over chicken in bag. Seal bag and turn to coat chicken. Place bag in a medium bowl; marinate in the refrigerator for 4 to 6 hours, turning bag occasionally.

2. Preheat broiler. In a large skillet heat 2 tablespoons of the coconut oil over medium heat. Add carrots, celery, and onion; cook for 6 to 8 minutes or until vegetables are tender, stirring occasionally. Add jalapeños; cook and stir for 1 minute more. Add undrained tomatoes and tomato sauce. Bring to boiling; reduce heat. Simmer, uncovered, about 5 minutes or until sauce thickens slightly.

3. Drain chicken, discarding marinade. Arrange chicken pieces in a single layer on the unheated rack of a broiler pan. Broil 5 to 6 inches from the heat for 8 to 10 minutes or until chicken is no longer pink, turning once halfway through broiling. Add cooked chicken pieces and the remaining ¼ cup coconut milk to tomato mixture in skillet. Cook for 1 to 2 minutes or until heated through. Remove from the heat; stir in garam masala.

4. Trim ends off zucchini. Using a julienne cutter, cut zucchini into long thin strips. In an extra-large skillet

heat the remaining 2 tablespoons coconut oil over medium-high heat. Add zucchini strips and black pepper. Cook and stir for 2 to 3 minutes or until zucchini is crisp-tender.

5. To serve, divide zucchini among four serving plates. Top with chicken mixture. Garnish with cilantro leaves.

RAS EL HANOUT CHICKEN THIGHS

PREP: 20 minutes COOK: 40 minutes MAKES: 4 servings

RAS EL HANOUT IS A COMPLEX AND EXOTIC MORROCAN SPICE MIXTURE. THE PHRASE MEANS "HEAD OF THE SHOP" IN ARABIC, WHICH IMPLIES THAT IT IS A UNIQUE BLEND OF THE BEST SPICES THE SPICE SELLER HAS TO OFFER. THERE'S NO SET RECIPE FOR RAS EL HANOUT, BUT IT OFTEN CONTAINS SOME BLEND OF GINGER, ANISE, CINNAMON, NUTMEG, PEPPERCORNS, CLOVES, CARDAMOM, DRIED FLOWERS (SUCH AS LAVENDER AND ROSE), NIGELLA, MACE, GALANGAL, AND TURMERIC.

- 1 tablespoon ground cumin
- 2 teaspoons ground ginger
- 1½ teaspoons black pepper
- 1½ teaspoons ground cinnamon
- 1 teaspoon ground coriander
- 1 teaspoon cayenne pepper
- 1 teaspoon ground allspice
- ½ teaspoon ground cloves
- ¼ teaspoon ground nutmeg
- 1 teaspoon saffron threads (optional)
- 4 tablespoons unrefined coconut oil
- 8 bone-in chicken thighs
- 1 8-ounce package fresh mushrooms, sliced
- 1 cup chopped onion
- 1 cup chopped red, yellow, or green sweet pepper (1 large)
- 4 roma tomatoes, cored, seeded, and chopped
- 4 cloves garlic, minced
- 2 13.5-ounce cans natural coconut milk (such as Nature's Way)
- 3 to 4 tablespoons fresh lime juice
- ¼ cup finely snipped fresh cilantro

1. For the ras el hanout, in medium mortar or small bowl combine the cumin, ginger, black pepper, cinnamon, coriander, cayenne pepper, allspice, cloves, nutmeg, and, if desired, saffron. Grind with a pestle or stir with a spoon to mix well. Set aside.

2. In an extra-large skillet heat 2 tablespoons of the coconut oil over medium heat. Sprinkle chicken thighs with 1 tablespoon of the ras el hanout. Add chicken to skillet; cook for 5 to 6 minutes or until browned, turning once halfway through cooking. Remove chicken from skillet; keep warm.

3. In the same skillet heat the remaining 2 tablespoons coconut oil over medium heat. Add mushrooms, onion, sweet pepper, tomatoes, and garlic. Cook and stir about 5 minutes or until vegetables are tender. Stir in coconut milk, lime juice, and 1 tablespoon of the ras el hanout. Return chicken to skillet. Bring to boiling; reduce heat. Simmer, covered, about 30 minutes or until chicken is tender (175°F).

4. Serve chicken, vegetables, and sauce in bowls. Garnish with cilantro.

Note: Store leftover Ras el Hanout in a covered container for up to 1 month.

STAR FRUIT ADOBO CHICKEN THIGHS OVER BRAISED SPINACH

PREP: 40 minutes MARINATE: 4 to 8 hours COOK: 45 minutes MAKES: 4 servings

IF NECESSARY, PAT THE CHICKEN DRY WITH A PAPER TOWEL AFTER IT COMES OUT OF THE MARINADE BEFORE BROWNING IT IN THE SKILLET. ANY LIQUID LEFT ON THE MEAT WILL SPATTER IN THE HOT OIL.

8 bone-in chicken thighs (1½ to 2 pounds), skinned

¾ cup white or cider vinegar

¾ cup fresh orange juice

½ cup water

¼ cup chopped onion

¼ cup snipped fresh cilantro

4 cloves garlic, minced

½ teaspoon black pepper

1 tablespoon olive oil

1 star fruit (carambola), sliced

1 cup Chicken Bone Broth (see recipe) or no-salt-added chicken broth

2 9-ounce packages fresh spinach leaves

Fresh cilantro leaves (optional)

1. Place chicken in a stainless-steel or enamel Dutch oven; set aside. In a medium bowl combine vinegar, orange juice, the water, onion, ¼ cup snipped cilantro, garlic, and pepper; pour over chicken. Cover and marinate in the refrigerator for 4 to 8 hours.

2. Bring chicken mixture in Dutch oven to boiling over medium-high heat; reduce heat. Cover and simmer for 35 to 40 minutes or until chicken is no longer pink (175°F).

3. In an extra-large skillet heat oil over medium-high heat. With tongs, remove chicken from Dutch oven, shaking gently so cooking liquid drips off; reserve cooking liquid. Brown the chicken on all sides, turning frequently to brown evenly.

4. Meanwhile, for sauce, strain cooking liquid; return to Dutch oven. Bring to boiling. Boil about 4 minutes to reduce and thicken slightly; add star fruit; boil for 1 minute more. Return chicken to the sauce in Dutch oven. Remove from heat; cover to keep warm.

5. Wipe out the skillet. Pour Chicken Bone Broth into skillet. Bring to boiling over medium-high heat; stir in spinach. Reduce heat; simmer for 1 to 2 minutes or until spinach is just wilted, stirring constantly. Using a slotted spoon, transfer spinach to a serving platter. Top with chicken and sauce. If desired, sprinkle with cilantro leaves.

CHICKEN-POBLANO CABBAGE TACOS WITH CHIPOTLE MAYO

PREP: 25 minutes BAKE: 40 minutes MAKES: 4 servings

SERVE THESE MESSY-BUT-TASTY TACOS WITH A FORK TO RETRIEVE ANY OF THE FILLING THAT HAPPENS TO FALL OUT OF THE CABBAGE LEAF WHILE YOU'RE EATING IT.

1 tablespoon olive oil

2 poblano chiles, seeded (if desired) and chopped (see tip)

½ cup chopped onion

3 cloves garlic, minced

1 tablespoon salt-free chili powder

2 teaspoons ground cumin

½ teaspoon black pepper

1 8-ounce can no-salt-added tomato sauce

¾ cup Chicken Bone Broth (see recipe) or no-salt-added chicken broth

1 teaspoon dried Mexican oregano, crushed

1 to 1½ pounds skinless, boneless chicken thighs

10 to 12 medium to large cabbage leaves

Chipotle Paleo Mayo (see recipe)

1. Preheat oven to 350°F. In a large ovenproof skillet heat oil over medium-high heat. Add poblano chiles, onion, and garlic; cook and stir for 2 minutes. Stir in chili powder, cumin, and black pepper; cook and stir for 1 minute more (if necessary, reduce heat to prevent spices from burning).

2. Add tomato sauce, Chicken Bone Broth, and oregano to skillet. Bring to boiling. Carefully place chicken thighs in the tomato mixture. Cover skillet with lid. Bake about 40

minutes or until chicken is tender (175°F), turning chicken once halfway.

3. Remove chicken from skillet; cool slightly. Using two forks, shred chicken into bite-size pieces. Stir shredded chicken into tomato mixture in skillet.

4. To serve, spoon chicken mixture into cabbage leaves; top with Chipotle Paleo Mayo.

CHICKEN STEW WITH BABY CARROTS AND BOK CHOY

PREP: 15 minutes COOK: 24 minutes STAND: 2 minutes MAKES: 4 servings

BABY BOK CHOY IS VERY DELICATE AND CAN GET OVERCOOKED IN A FLASH. TO KEEP IT CRISP AND FRESH-TASTING—NOT WILTED AND SOGGY—BE SURE IT STEAMS IN THE COVERED HOT POT (OFF THE HEAT) FOR NO MORE THAN 2 MINUTES BEFORE YOU SERVE THE STEW.

- 2 tablespoons olive oil
- 1 leek, sliced (white and light green parts)
- 4 cups Chicken Bone Broth (see recipe) or no-salt-added chicken broth
- 1 cup dry white wine
- 1 tablespoon Dijon-Style Mustard (see recipe)
- ½ teaspoon black pepper
- 1 sprig fresh thyme
- 1¼ pounds skinless, boneless chicken thighs, cut into 1-inch pieces
- 8 ounces baby carrots with tops, scrubbed, trimmed, and halved lengthwise, or 2 medium carrots, bias-sliced
- 2 teaspoons finely shredded lemon peel (set aside)
- 1 tablespoon fresh lemon juice
- 2 heads baby bok choy
- ½ teaspoon snipped fresh thyme

1. In a large saucepan heat 1 tablespoon of the olive oil over medium heat. Cook leek in hot oil for 3 to 4 minutes or until wilted. Add Chicken Bone Broth, wine, Dijon-Style Mustard, ¼ teaspoon of the pepper, and thyme sprig. Bring to boiling; reduce heat. Cook for 10

to 12 minutes or until liquid is reduced by about one-third. Discard thyme sprig.

2. Meanwhile, in a Dutch oven heat the remaining 1 tablespoon olive oil over medium-high heat. Sprinkle chicken with the remaining ¼ teaspoon pepper. Cook in hot oil about 3 minutes or until browned, stirring occasionally. Drain fat if necessary. Carefully add the reduced broth mixture to pot, scraping up any brown bits; add carrots. Bring to boiling; reduce heat. Simmer, uncovered, for 8 to 10 minutes or just until carrots are tender. Stir in lemon juice. Cut bok choy in half lengthwise. (If bok choy heads are large, cut into quarters.) Place bok choy on top of chicken in pot. Cover and remove from heat; let stand for 2 minutes.

3. Ladle stew into shallow bowls. Sprinkle with lemon peel and snipped thyme.

CASHEW-ORANGE CHICKEN AND SWEET PEPPER STIR-FRY IN LETTUCE WRAPS

START TO FINISH: 45 minutes MAKES: 4 to 6 servings

YOU WILL FIND TWO TYPES OF COCONUT OIL ON THE
SHELVES—REFINED AND EXTRA VIRGIN, OR UNREFINED.
AS THE NAME IMPLIES, EXTRA VIRGIN COCONUT OIL IS
FROM THE FIRST PRESSING OF THE FRESH, RAW
COCONUT. IT IS ALWAYS THE BETTER CHOICE WHEN
YOU ARE COOKING OVER MEDIUM OR MEDIUM-HIGH
HEAT. REFINED COCONUT OIL HAS A HIGHER SMOKE
POINT, SO USE IT ONLY WHEN YOU ARE COOKING OVER
HIGH HEAT.

1 tablespoon refined coconut oil

1½ to 2 pounds skinless, boneless chicken thighs, cut into thin bite-size strips

3 red, orange, and/or yellow sweet peppers, stemmed, seeded, and thinly sliced into bite-size strips

1 red onion, halved lengthwise and thinly sliced

1 teaspoon finely shredded orange peel (set aside)

½ cup fresh orange juice

1 tablespoon minced fresh ginger

3 cloves garlic, minced

1 cup unsalted raw cashews, toasted and coarsely chopped (see tip)

½ cup sliced green scallions (4)

8 to 10 butter or iceberg lettuce leaves

1. In a wok or large skillet heat the coconut oil over high heat. Add chicken; cook and stir for 2 minutes. Add peppers and onion; cook and stir for 2 to 3 minutes or

until vegetables just start to soften. Remove the chicken and vegetables from the wok; keep warm.

2. Wipe out wok with paper towel. Add the orange juice to the wok. Cook about 3 minutes or until juice boils and reduces slightly. Add ginger and garlic. Cook and stir for 1 minute. Return the chicken and pepper mixture to the wok. Stir in orange peel, cashews, and scallions. Serve stir-fry on lettuce leaves.

VIETNAMESE COCONUT-LEMONGRASS CHICKEN

START TO FINISH: 30 minutes MAKES: 4 servings

THIS QUICK COCONUT CURRY CAN BE ON THE TABLE IN 30 MINUTES FROM THE TIME YOU START CHOPPING, MAKING IT AN IDEAL MEAL FOR A BUSY WEEKNIGHT.

- 1 tablespoon unrefined coconut oil
- 4 stalks lemongrass (pale parts only)
- 1 3.2-ounce package oyster mushrooms, chopped
- 1 large onion, thinly sliced, rings halved
- 1 fresh jalapeño, seeded and finely chopped (see tip)
- 2 tablespoons minced fresh ginger
- 3 cloves garlic minced
- 1½ pounds skinless, boneless chicken thighs, thinly sliced and cut into bite-size pieces
- ½ cup natural coconut milk (such as Nature's Way)
- ½ cup Chicken Bone Broth (see recipe) or no-salt-added chicken broth
- 1 tablespoon salt-free red curry powder
- ½ teaspoon black pepper
- ½ cup snipped fresh basil leaves
- 2 tablespoons fresh lime juice
- Unsweetened shaved coconut (optional)

1. In an extra-large skillet heat coconut oil over medium heat. Add lemongrass; cook and stir for 1 minute. Add mushrooms, onion, jalapeño, ginger, and garlic; cook and stir for 2 minutes or until onion is just tender. Add chicken; cook about 3 minutes or until chicken is cooked through.

2. In a small bowl combine coconut milk, Chicken Bone Broth, curry powder, and black pepper. Add to chicken mixture in skillet; cook for 1 minute or until the liquid has slightly thickened. Remove from heat; stir in fresh basil and lime juice. If desired, sprinkle servings with coconut.

GRILLED CHICKEN AND APPLE ESCAROLE SALAD

PREP: 30 minutes GRILL: 12 minutes MAKES: 4 servings

IF YOU LIKE A SWEETER APPLE, GO WITH HONEYCRISP. IF YOU LIKE A TART APPLE, USE GRANNY SMITH—OR, FOR BALANCE, TRY A MIX OF THE TWO VARIETIES.

3 medium Honeycrisp or Granny Smith apples

4 teaspoons extra virgin olive oil

½ cup finely chopped shallots

2 tablespoons snipped fresh parsley

1 tablespoon poultry seasoning

3 to 4 heads escarole, quartered

1 pound ground chicken or turkey breast

⅓ cup chopped toasted hazelnuts*

⅓ cup Classic French Vinaigrette (see recipe)

1. Halve and core apples. Peel and finely chop 1 of the apples. In a medium skillet heat 1 teaspoon of the olive oil over medium heat. Add chopped apple and shallots; cook until tender. Stir in parsley and poultry seasoning. Set aside to cool.

2. Meanwhile, core the remaining 2 apples and cut into wedges. Brush cut sides of apple wedges and escarole with the remaining olive oil. In a large bowl combine chicken and the cooled apple mixture. Divide into eight portions; shape each portion into a 2-inch-diameter patty.

3. For a charcoal or gas grill, place chicken patties and apple wedges on a grill rack directly over medium heat.

Cover and grill for 10 minutes, turning once halfway through grilling. Add escarole, cut sides down. Cover and grill for 2 to 4 minutes or until escarole is lightly charred, apples are tender, and chicken patties are done (165°F).

4. Coarsely chop escarole. Divide escarole among four serving plates. Top with chicken patties, apple slices, and hazelnuts. Drizzle with Classic French Vinaigrette.

*Tip: To toast hazelnuts, preheat oven to 350°F. Spread nuts in a single layer in a shallow baking pan. Bake for 8 to 10 minutes or until lightly toasted, stirring once to toast evenly. Cool nuts slightly. Place the warm nuts on a clean kitchen towel; rub with the towel to remove the loose skins.

TUSCAN CHICKEN SOUP WITH KALE RIBBONS

PREP: 15 minutes COOK: 20 minutes MAKES: 4 to 6 servings

A SPOONFUL OF PESTO—YOUR CHOICE OF EITHER BASIL OR ARUGULA—ADDS GREAT TASTE TO THIS SAVORY SOUP SEASONED WITH SALT-FREE POULTRY SEASONING. TO KEEP THE KALE RIBBONS BRIGHT GREEN AND AS FULL OF NUTRIENTS AS POSSIBLE, COOK THEM ONLY UNTIL THEY WILT.

1 pound ground chicken

2 tablespoons no-salt-added poultry seasoning

1 teaspoon finely shredded lemon peel

1 tablespoon olive oil

1 cup chopped onion

½ cup chopped carrots

1 cup chopped celery

4 cloves garlic, sliced

4 cups Chicken Bone Broth (see recipe) or no-salt-added chicken broth

1 14.5-ounce can no-salt-added fire-roasted tomatoes, undrained

1 bunch Lacinato (Tuscan) kale, stems removed, cut into ribbons

2 tablespoons fresh lemon juice

1 teaspoon snipped fresh thyme

Basil or Arugula Pesto (see recipes)

1. In a medium bowl combine ground chicken, poultry seasoning, and lemon peel. Mix well.

2. In a Dutch oven heat olive oil over medium heat. Add chicken mixture, onion, carrots, and celery; cook for 5 to 8 minutes or until chicken is no longer pink, stirring with a wooden spoon to break up meat and adding garlic

slices the last 1 minute of cooking. Add Chicken Bone Broth and tomatoes. Bring to boiling; reduce heat. Cover and simmer for 15 minutes. Stir in kale, lemon juice, and thyme. Simmer, uncovered, about 5 minutes or until kale is just wilted.

3. To serve, ladle soup into serving bowls and top with Basil or Arugula Pesto.

CHICKEN LARB

THIS VERSION OF THE POPULAR THAI DISH OF HIGHLY SEASONED GROUND CHICKEN AND VEGETABLES SERVED IN LETTUCE LEAVES IS INCREDIBLY LIGHT AND FLAVORFUL—WITHOUT THE ADDITION OF THE SUGAR, SALT, AND FISH SAUCE (WHICH IS VERY HIGH IN SODIUM) THAT ARE TRADITIONALLY PART OF THE INGREDIENTS LIST. WITH GARLIC, THAI CHILES, LEMONGRASS, LIME PEEL, LIME JUICE, MINT, AND CILANTRO, YOU WON'T MISS THEM.

- 1 tablespoon refined coconut oil
- 2 pounds ground chicken (95% lean or ground breast)
- 8 ounces button mushrooms, finely chopped
- 1 cup finely chopped red onion
- 1 to 2 Thai chiles, seeded and finely chopped (see tip)
- 2 tablespoons minced garlic
- 2 tablespoons finely chopped lemongrass*
- ¼ teaspoon ground cloves
- ¼ teaspoon black pepper
- 1 tablespoon finely shredded lime peel
- ½ cup fresh lime juice
- ⅓ cup tightly packed fresh mint leaves, chopped
- ⅓ cup tightly packed fresh cilantro, chopped
- 1 head iceberg lettuce, separated into leaves

1. In an extra-large skillet heat coconut oil over medium-high heat. Add ground chicken, mushrooms, onion, chile(s), garlic, lemongrass, cloves, and black pepper. Cook for 8 to 10 minutes or until chicken is cooked through, stirring with a wooden spoon to break up meat

as it cooks. Drain if necessary. Transfer chicken mixture to an extra-large bowl. Let cool about 20 minutes or until slightly warmer than room temperature, stirring occasionally.

2. Stir lime peel, lime juice, mint, and cilantro into chicken mixture. Serve in lettuce leaves.

*Tip: To prepare the lemongrass, you'll need a sharp knife. Cut the woody stem off of the bottom of the stalk and the tough green blades at the top of the plant. Remove the two tough outer layers. You should have a piece of lemongrass that is about 6 inches long and pale yellow-white. Cut the stalk in half horizontally, then cut each half in half again. Slice each quarter of the stalk very thinly.

CHICKEN BURGERS WITH SZECHWAN CASHEW SAUCE

PREP: 30 minutes COOK: 5 minutes GRILL: 14 minutes MAKES: 4 servings

THE CHILI OIL MADE BY WARMING OLIVE OIL WITH CRUSHED RED PEPPER CAN BE USED IN OTHER WAYS AS WELL. USE IT TO SAUTÉ FRESH VEGETABLES—OR TOSS THEM WITH SOME CHILI OIL BEFORE ROASTING.

2 tablespoons olive oil

¼ teaspoon crushed red pepper

2 cups raw cashew pieces, toasted (see tip)

¼ cup olive oil

½ cup shredded zucchini

¼ cup finely chopped chives

2 cloves garlic, minced

2 teaspoons finely shredded lemon peel

2 teaspoons grated fresh ginger

1 pound ground chicken or turkey breast

SZECHWAN CASHEW SAUCE

1 tablespoon olive oil

2 tablespoons finely chopped scallions

1 tablespoon grated fresh ginger

1 teaspoon Chinese five-spice powder

1 teaspoon fresh lime juice

4 green leaf or butter lettuce leaves

1. For the chili oil, in a small saucepan combine the olive oil and the crushed red pepper. Warm over low heat for 5 minutes. Remove from heat; let cool.

2. For cashew butter, place cashews and 1 tablespoon of the olive oil in a blender. Cover and blend until creamy,

102

stopping to scrape down the sides as needed and adding additional olive oil, 1 tablespoon at a time, until the entire ¼ cup has been used and the butter is very soft; set aside.

3. In a large bowl combine the zucchini, chives, garlic, lemon peel, and the 2 teaspoons ginger. Add ground chicken; mix well. Shape chicken mixture into four ½-inch-thick patties.

4. For a charcoal or gas grill, place patties on the greased rack directly over medium heat. Cover and grill for 14 to 16 minutes or until done (165°F), turning once halfway through grilling.

5. Meanwhile, for the sauce, in a small skillet heat the olive oil over medium heat. Add the scallions and the 1 tablespoon ginger; cook over medium-low heat for 2 minutes or until scallions soften. Add ½ cup of the cashew butter (refrigerate remaining cashew butter for up to 1 week), chili oil, lime juice, and five-spice powder. Cook for 2 more minutes. Remove from heat.

6. Serve patties on the lettuce leaves. Drizzle with sauce.

TURKISH CHICKEN WRAPS

PREP: 25 minutes STAND: 15 minutes COOK: 8 minutes MAKES: 4 to 6 servings

"BAHARAT" SIMPLY MEANS "SPICE" IN ARABIC. AN ALL-PURPOSE SEASONING IN MIDDLE EASTERN CUISINE, IT IS OFTEN USED AS A RUB ON FISH, POULTRY, AND MEATS OR MIXED WITH OLIVE OIL AND USED AS A VEGETABLE MARINADE. THE COMBINATION OF WARM, SWEET SPICES SUCH AS CINNAMON, CUMIN, CORIANDER, CLOVES, AND PAPRIKA MAKES IT PARTICULARLY AROMATIC. THE ADDITION OF DRIED MINT IS A TURKISH TOUCH.

⅓ cup snipped unsulfured dried apricots

⅓ cup snipped dried figs

1 tablespoon unrefined coconut oil

1½ pounds ground chicken breast

3 cups sliced leeks (white and light green parts only) (3)

⅔ of a medium green and/or red sweet peppers, thinly sliced

2 tablespoons Baharat Seasoning (see recipe, below)

2 cloves garlic, minced

1 cup chopped, seeded tomatoes (2 medium)

1 cup chopped, seeded cucumber (½ of a medium)

½ cup chopped shelled unsalted pistachios, toasted (see tip)

¼ cup snipped fresh mint

¼ cup snipped fresh parsley

8 to 12 large butterhead or Bibb lettuce leaves

1. Place apricots and figs in a small bowl. Add ⅔ cup boiling water; let stand for 15 minutes. Drain, reserving ½ cup of the liquid.

2. Meanwhile, in an extra-large skillet heat coconut oil over medium heat. Add ground chicken; cook for 3 minutes,

stirring with a wooden spoon to break up meat as it cooks. Add leeks, sweet pepper, Baharat Seasoning, and garlic; cook and stir about 3 minutes or until chicken is done and pepper is just tender. Add apricots, figs, reserved liquid, tomatoes, and cucumber. Cook and stir about 2 minutes or until tomatoes and cucumber just start to break down. Stir in pistachios, mint, and parsley.

3. Serve chicken and vegetables in lettuce leaves.

Baharat Seasoning: In a small bowl combine 2 tablespoons sweet paprika; 1 tablespoon black pepper; 2 teaspoons dried mint, finely crushed; 2 teaspoons ground cumin; 2 teaspoons ground coriander; 2 teaspoons ground cinnamon; 2 teaspoons ground cloves; 1 teaspoon ground nutmeg; and 1 teaspoon ground cardamom. Store in a tightly sealed container at room temperature. Makes about ½ cup.

SPANISH CORNISH HENS

PREP: 10 minutes BAKE: 30 minutes BROIL: 6 minutes MAKES: 2 to 3 servings

THIS RECIPE COULD NOT BE EASIER—AND THE RESULTS ARE ABSOLUTELY AMAZING. COPIOUS AMOUNTS OF SMOKED PAPRIKA, GARLIC, AND LEMON GIVE THESE DIMINUTIVE BIRDS BIG FLAVOR.

2 1½-pound Cornish hens, thawed if frozen

1 tablespoon olive oil

6 cloves garlic, chopped

2 to 3 tablespoons smoked sweet paprika

¼ to ½ teaspoon cayenne pepper (optional)

2 lemons, quartered

2 tablespoons snipped fresh parsley (optional)

1. Preheat oven to 375°F. To quarter the game hens, use kitchen shears or a sharp knife to cut along both sides of the narrow backbone. Butterfly the bird open and cut the hen in half through the breastbone. Remove the hind-quarters by cutting through the skin and meat that separates the thighs from the breast. Keep the wing and breast intact. Rub olive oil over Cornish hen pieces. Sprinkle with chopped garlic.

2. Place the hen pieces, skin sides up, in an extra-large oven-going skillet. Sprinkle with smoked paprika and cayenne. Squeeze the lemon quarters over the hens; add lemon quarters to the skillet. Turn hen pieces skin sides down in the pan. Cover and bake for 30 minutes. Remove skillet from oven.

3. Preheat broiler. Using tongs, turn the pieces. Adjust oven rack. Broil 4 to 5 inches from the heat for 6 to 8 minutes until skin is browned and hens are done (175°F). Drizzle with pan juices. If desired, sprinkle with parsley.

PISTACHIO-ROASTED CORNISH HENS WITH ARUGULA, APRICOT, AND FENNEL SALAD

PREP: 30 minutes CHILL: 2 to 12 hours ROAST: 50 minutes STAND: 10 minutes
MAKES: 8 servings

A PISTACHIO PESTO MADE WITH PARSLEY, THYME, GARLIC, ORANGE PEEL, ORANGE JUICE, AND OLIVE OIL IS TUCKED UNDER THE SKIN OF EACH BIRD BEFORE MARINATING.

- 4 20- to 24-ounce Cornish game hens
- 3 cups raw pistachio nuts
- 2 tablespoons snipped fresh Italian (flat-leaf) parsley
- 1 tablespoon snipped thyme
- 1 large clove garlic, minced
- 2 teaspoons finely shredded orange peel
- 2 tablespoons fresh orange juice
- ¾ cup olive oil
- 2 large onions, thinly sliced
- ½ cup fresh orange juice
- 2 tablespoons fresh lemon juice
- ¼ teaspoon freshly ground black pepper
- ¼ teaspoon dry mustard
- 2 5-ounce packages arugula
- 1 large bulb fennel, thinly shaved
- 2 tablespoons snipped fennel fronds
- 4 apricots, pitted and cut into thin wedges

1. Rinse inside cavities of Cornish game hens. Tie legs together with 100%-cotton kitchen string. Tuck wings under bodies; set aside.

2. In a food processor or blender combine pistachios, parsley, thyme, garlic, orange peel, and orange juice. Process until coarse paste forms. With processor running, add ¼ cup of the olive oil in a slow, steady stream.

3. Using fingers, loosen skin on the breast side of a hen to make a pocket. Spread one-fourth of the pistachio mixture evenly under the skin. Repeat with remaining hens and pistachio mixture. Spread sliced onions over bottom of roasting pan; place hens, breast sides up, on top of onions. Cover and refrigerate for 2 to 12 hours.

4. Preheat oven to 425°F. Roast hens for 30 to 35 minutes or until an instant-read thermometer inserted in an inside thigh muscle registers 175°F.

5. Meanwhile, for dressing, in a small bowl combine orange juice, lemon juice, pepper, and mustard. Mix well. Add the remaining ½ cup olive oil in a slow steady stream, whisking constantly.

6. For salad, in a large bowl combine arugula, fennel, fennel fronds, and apricots. Drizzle lightly with dressing; toss well. Reserve additional dressing for another purpose.

7. Remove hens from oven; tent loosely with foil and let stand 10 minutes. To serve, divide the salad evenly among eight serving plates. Cut hens in half lengthwise; place hen halves on salads. Serve immediately.

DUCK BREAST WITH POMEGRANATE AND JICAMA SALAD

PREP: 15 minutes COOK: 15 minutes MAKES: 4 servings

CUTTING A DIAMOND PATTERN INTO THE FAT OF THE DUCK BREASTS ALLOWS THE FAT TO RENDER OUT AS THE GARAM MASALA-SEASONED BREASTS COOK. THE DRIPPINGS ARE COMBINED WITH JICAMA, POMEGRANATE SEEDS, ORANGE JUICE, AND BEEF BROTH AND TOSSED WITH PEPPERY GREENS TO WILT THEM JUST SLIGHTLY.

4 boneless Muscovy duck breasts (about 1½ to 2 pounds total)

1 tablespoon garam masala

1 tablespoon unrefined coconut oil

2 cups diced, peeled jicama

½ cup pomegranate seeds

¼ cup fresh orange juice

¼ cup Beef Bone Broth (see recipe) or no-salt-added beef broth

3 cups watercress, stems removed

3 cups torn frisée and/or thinly sliced Belgian endive

1. With a sharp knife, make shallow cuts in diamond patterns into the fat of duck breasts at 1-inch intervals. Sprinkle both sides of the breast halves with the garam masala. Heat an extra-large skillet over medium heat. Melt the coconut oil in the hot skillet. Place breast halves, skin sides down, in the skillet. Cook for 8 minutes with the skin sides down, being careful not to brown too quickly (reduce heat if necessary). Turn duck

breasts over; cook for 5 to 6 minutes more or until an instant-read thermometer inserted into breast halves registers 145°F for medium. Remove breast halves, reserving drippings in a skillet; cover with foil to keep warm.

2. For dressing, add jicama to drippings in skillet; cook and stir for 2 minutes over medium heat. Add pomegranate seeds, orange juice, and Beef Bone Broth to skillet. Bring to boiling; immediately remove from heat.

3. For salad, in a large bowl combine watercress and frisée. Pour hot dressing over greens; toss to coat.

4. Divide salad among four dinner plates. Thinly slice the duck breasts and arrange on salads.

HEIRLOOM TOMATO AND WATERMELON SALAD WITH PINK PEPPERCORN DRIZZLE

START TO FINISH: 30 minutes MAKES: 6 servings PHOTO

THIS IS SUMMER IN A BOWL—JUICY RIPE HEIRLOOM TOMATOES AND WATERMELON. USING A MIX OF HEIRLOOM TOMATOES—WHATEVER YOU'RE GROWING IN YOUR GARDEN, GET IN YOUR CSA BOX, OR BUY AT THE FARMER'S MARKET—WILL MAKE A BEAUTIFUL PRESENTATION.

- 1 miniature seedless watermelon (4 to 4½ pounds)
- 4 large heirloom tomatoes
- ¼ of a red onion, cut into paper-thin slivers
- ¼ cup loosely packed fresh mint leaves
- ¼ cup basil chiffonade*
- ¼ cup olive oil
- 2 tablespoons fresh lemon juice
- 1½ teaspoons pink peppercorns

1. Remove rind from watermelon; cut melon into 1-inch chunks. Stem and core tomatoes; cut into wedges. On a large serving platter or in a large serving bowl combine watermelon chunks and tomato wedges; toss to combine. Sprinkle with onion, mint, and basil chiffonade.

112

2. For dressing, in a small jar with a tight-fitting lid combine olive oil, lemon juice, and peppercorns. Cover and shake vigorously to combine. Drizzle over tomato-watermelon salad. Serve at room temperature.

*Note: For a chiffonade, stack the basil leaves on top of one another and roll up tightly. Thinly slice the roll, then separate the basil into thin ribbons.

Lightning Source UK Ltd.
Milton Keynes UK
UKHW020641180621
385739UK00011B/585